HEALING CANCER
WITH
QIGONG

HEALING CANCER
WITH
QIGONG

One man's search for healing and love in curing his cancer with
complementary therapy

SAT HON

Books and Essays by Sat Hon:

Taoist Qigong For Health and Vitality, Shambhala Press, 2003

Soul & Spirit of Tea, 21 Tea-inspired Essays for the Early Twenty-first Century, edited by
Phil Cousineau & Scott Chamberlin Hoyt,
with Sat Hon and 19 contributors.

Published by Ancient Taoist Practice Society, Inc.
(A Non-profit educational Incorporation.)

The author of this book does not give out medical advice or prescribe the use of any technique as a form of treatment for physical, emotional, or medical problems without the advice of a qualified medical professionals. It is not meant to replace your treatment with your health care providers nor should you stop taking any medications. Always seek the advice of a medical doctor in regard to any physical, psychological or emotional condition. In the event you apply any of the information in this book for yourself, the author and the publisher assume no responsibility for your actions.

To my wife who loves me with fearless devotion,
and to my daughters, Singha, Jimei and Lingji,
who gave me the divine gift of life,
a mandate to seek *real* help.

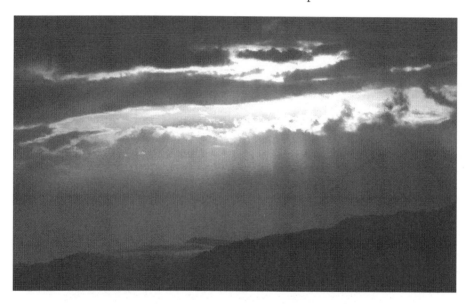

BHAGAVAD GITA

"Be wise in matters of death and life. See in this epic battle presented by chance a gateway toward liberation. For certain is death that all that's born, for sure is birth to all that dies and for this, you have no cause to regret. Likewise, recognize this struggle as propelled by the karmic tide. Embrace ecstasy and agony, gain and loss, victory and defeat with equanimity, and then brace yourself ready for the fight. So will you bring no evil onto yourself"

CONTENTS

FOREWARD

There are three perspectives that I bring with me as I write this foreward. First, I am a Western trained medical practitioner, specializing in dermatology, in private practice with an appointment as a Clinical Associate Professor at Brown University. I am a lifelong student. My curiosity and constant search for knowledge led me to a workshop on Medical Qigong led by Master Hon. One thing that initially attracted me to qigong was the inside/outside parallel that was an integral to my specialty. The skin as the largest organ can reflect the health of a person, both physically and mentally. This opened a door for my mind to explore the possibility, and then realize the truth of this Eastern wisdom. Master Hon so eloquently describes qigong as a movement symphony. This practice is rooted in shamanic dance and is able to refine and affect the well-being of the practitioner. As a physician, I acknowledge the strength and wisdom of bridging Western and Eastern perspectives to health.

Secondly, I had been a caregiver to my late husband for his four-year battle with cancer. I came to the practice of qigong after his death and it has been invaluable in aiding me with the grief and loss, and is so now as I move to the next phase of my life. I can look back at my role as a caregiver and see where qigong would have been a support for me, and for my husband had he been receptive during that time. There was only a minimal complementary medicine program where my husband received treatment. There was the occasional Reiki practitioner who would come through the infusion center to offer chair side treatments, and the pet therapy dog. My husband was only receptive to the latter. In some ways I think his stubbornness served him well on his journey and kept his spirit rooted in his personal battle. Yet I think there could have been some softening on the battlefield had been more receptive. The practice of qigong has much more to offer than merely coping with illness. It can be a life-affirming practice and its power can propel one from loss to personal growth, as it has for me.

Looking back to my four years as caregiver to a cancer patient, I realize in retrospect that I had unconsciously adopted a type of moving meditation in my passion for running. While at the cancer treatment center, during my husband's frequent infusion sessions, I would climb up and down 15 flights of stairs several times a day in lieu of my usual running routine. It was a much needed break from the hours sitting in the infusion room. Focusing on one step at a time helped to clear and calm my mind. This was part of my ongoing healing as a caregiver of a terminally ill patient and a realization that came to me much later.

Thirdly, it is my privilege to be a fledgling student of my Sifu, Master Hon. Although my time in practice is short compared to many of his students, I am here to acknowledge the transformative power of qigong. The voice you hear in my words reflects all that history, yet my practice of qigong brings me change and growth. Integrating qigong, spirituality, and meditation are not merely a powerful combination for dealing with illness but are essential tools for living a full life.

I have been honored to have been asked to write a foreward for this book which can be viewed on several levels--the personal and heroic journey of a cancer patient, and the transmission of the healing of qigong from a compassionate and wise teacher. This is a book written from the heart. This is a book of empowerment. The honesty sings out from the tale of courage, recovery and love.

Just as this story is woven of many colorful and personal threads, the journey of cancer treatment is multilayered and multi personal. It is not a straight path but a roller coaster with the family, friends, coworkers, the medical team and complementary healers along for the ride. The impact of a cancer diagnosis is far reaching; the healing needs to be, as well. The caregivers, the family members and all those within the circle of impact may be inadvertently overlooked as the focus rightly remains on the front line, the patient. The value of complementary healing for these others is also great. Meditation and qigong can heal the spirit that is wounded by another's cancer diagnosis and help maintain the health of the caregiver. The mind-body connection is so evident here. The partnering of Eastern and Western healing is a boon to all.

In the deep silences that accompany us on our journey through life we may perceive a glimpse of our true self. Some of the silences will be powerfully uplifting, and others can be oppressively heavy like the weight of hearing a cancer diagnosis so like a thunderbolt. Acknowledging this power may allow you to see how the dynamic of the mind-body paradigm can be tapped to promote well-being. This book can instruct you as you take part in your own healing.

It is likely that you are reading this book because you either have cancer or are a loved one or caregiver of a person with cancer. As a very old saying goes, "When the student is ready, the teacher will appear." It is my wish for you that the lessons in this book will empower you on your journey.

—Marla Angermeier, MD
16 October 2014

INTRODUCTION

The book you are holding in your hands is at once amazing, inspiring and transformative.

This is a true story told by Sat Hon, a present day Tai Chi and Qigong master. It begins when, as a well known healer in his own right, Sat Hon discovered he was ill with cancer. This first account is stark and moving. Failing at first to cure himself with Chinese traditional techniques of acupuncture and diet, he finally succumbed to the pleas of his children and turned to Western medicine—chemotherapy as directed by two Integrative Oncologists—Dr. M and Dr G. Probably aided by an initial traditional cleansing, the chemotherapy worked quickly and before long, he was free of cancer cells.

But this was just the beginning of his cure.

At this point in the account Sat Hon acquaints the reader with a condensed but quite forceful history of TCM – traditional Chinese medicine from the Taoist and Buddhist practices. The combined effect of Western medicine and ancient Chinese training is clearly demonstrated by his own complete recovery.

Sat Hon is in his own person a product of the twin traditions of Chinese and Western culture. At the age of 13 he arrived with his family in New York's Chinatown coming from main land China by way of Hong Kong. After high school he was awarded a full scholarship at Princeton University where he immersed himself in neuroscience and academic studies. He also began his career there as a part time Qigong teacher—a handy way to make additional money in his student years. After graduation he pursued studies in choreography in Connecticut before settling down as a Tai Chi and Qigong teacher in New York City. During the next years he and his wife Janet began a family—they have three daughters. He also has returned to main land China several times to complete his studies in acupuncture and TCM.

This book was written by a practitioner with first hand experience of Western medicine and a thorough knowledge of traditional Chinese practices. This, along with the incomparable motivation of saving his own life, made it possible for Sat Hon to achieve the realizations that are at the heart of his story.

Throughout these pages Sat Hon often refers to Alchemy. Here we should understand that it means a 'system of profound transformation'. Though never articulated, I think that we should also understand that Sat Hon is himself the Alchemist.

I have seen his work in traditional Chinese calligraphy and his translations of ancient Taoist poetry into English. I have also been one of his Qigong students for the past eighteen years. I knew him when he was going back to China to complete his CTM and acupuncture training. Also, I have known him during his illness and recovery. In addition we have to date completed two movement/ music collaborations—*Chaotic Harmony* and *Tai Chi on 23rd Street*.

So it is with great pleasure that I have written this introduction for Sat Hon—the Taoist/Buddhist practitioner, the Qigong/Tai Chi teacher and my friend.

—Phillip Glass

PREFACE

Complementary Therapy is the central theme that runs throughout this whole book. The power of this approach, in essence, integrates Traditional Chinese Medicine's internal metaphorical depiction of the human anatomy, Qigong's yogic-like shamanic sacred movement, and Buddhism's psychology and meditation. Complementary Therapy is a singular unified frontal assault on the ravaging cancer burning within. It was a life-saver for me along side standard Western medical treatments.

Like other cancer recovery memoirs my narrative is very personal and intended to inspire hope for others caught in the plight and fight against this insidious foe. However, unlike most cancer stories you may hear a Zen-like tone with ties to the ancient chants of shamans whose presence pierces through the annals of time to vibrate the marrow of the soul and cleanse us of dark entity possessions. It is then that you, the reader, may suddenly realize that cancer has always co-existed on the flip-side of normal biology. Cancer has evolved along a most perilous path, and with parasitic stealth flourishes on the stuff of our everyday lives—our drugs, poisonous chemicals, psychological stress and environmental pollution. Oh, how cancer thrives in this environment!

In a mirror-like parallel universe, once cancer has acquired a toe-hold in the body, it will tirelessly change its biological surroundings to suit its needs with maniacal efficiency and with rabid reproduction poison the host's circulation system with cancerous agents, induce it to grow extra blood vessel for the tumors, and as cancer thrives in insulin secretions, it will alter the eating habits of the host to ingest copious amounts of sugar in the form of cookies, ice cream or soft drinks. Think of all the changes that the host's body has undertaken in order for cancer to firmly establish itself. In truth, unlike an infection which invades from the outside, cancer is like being possessed from within by one's own evil twin—a cellular mutation of one's DNA. So healing and curing cancer is more akin to exorcism than to just killing a foreign invader. Therefore, cancer demands a total shift in the therapeutic paradigm of cancer treatment protocol, a complete approach of body, mind and spirit.

You may have posed this argument to your oncologist: Should you use a complementary approach or methods strictly consisting of Western medical technology: chemotherapy, radiation, surgery and experimental drugs? In most cases, their answer would be: "I don't know what other complementary treatments would be appropriate with the standard FDA approved medical procedures. It's not within the scope of my medical training." So true, oncologists are scientists in the field of pathology and they are certainly not the shaman and alchemist of old. Hence, in the following pages, I will serve as a guide along this shamanic quest in search of the exorcism of the evil twin within called "cancer". May my words and experience help you in your trials and tribulations. May your struggle be victorious.

PROLOGUE

How to describe the suffering, loneliness and alienation of my own journey of healing? Is it possible to recount the many hues of despair, the tones of rejoice and the deep silence that accompanied me? There were moments where I felt as if I was treading in the airless black space outside a space station with the Earth, a swirling green marble, beneath me.

When one unspools a strand of silk from a cocoon, the filament is so fine and delicate that the slightest tug will break the thread. One must therefore unwind the silk with breathless stealth as if moving in slow motion without the slightest abruptness. For hours, one spins and wraps the silk on a small bamboo wheel then suddenly without warning the naked pupae of the silk moth tumbles out. It dawns on one quite astonishing that the whole cocoon is composed of a single continuous thread. One must therefore, gently place the exposed pupae still in its translucent shell in a box with soft cotton and house it in your bosom to keep it warm. Within a few days the silk moth emerges with wings still brimming with sap, unfurling its furry antennas as it flutters out. Perchance this might be the way to write this book and unwind the pain, sorrow and joy that wrapped around my heart and let the words flutter out.

My journey would have been short had I not paid heed the pleas of my daughters. They compelled me to relinquish my initial alternative cancer treatment comprised of methods I was familiar with as a Chinese doctor: diet, fasting, nutritional supplements/herbs, acupuncture, qigong, meditation and drastic lifestyle changes. I was stubborn in my attempt to heal myself without standard chemotherapy and so sure that my alternative treatments could cure my cancer that I did not even bother to consult an oncologist. In hindsight, I realize that my fear of the alien territory of standard oncological treatment drove my obstinacy. So instead I clung to the familiar techniques that had been effective in my own practice of healing others.

It was quite convenient that the Internet is replete with anecdotes of spontaneous healing through nothing more than eating apple seeds or by converting to extreme vegetarianism. Even though most of these tales are scientifically unsubstantiated, for a drowning man in the throes of panic, any straw would do. I found myself completely lost in the wilderness of cancer healing, surrounded by advisors who could only agree with my chosen direction. Caught in a bubble of deluded optimism, I can still distinctively recall writing in my journal that cancer is not a disease, but a life out of balance. Ah, how fatally mistaken was I!

Fortunately, through the incessant pleas and finally blackmail by my daughters (who love me to distraction); I reluctantly agreed to consult with an integrative oncologist. Privately, I had already discarded any hope that such an oncologist would be able to contribute anything to my healing, but I made an appointment in order to satisfy my daughters' demands.

The trajectory of my healing path was littered with missteps, results of my own arrogance and pigheaded willfulness, inflicting great pain and anguish on my loved ones. However, this is a story of grace and spectacular redemption having ultimately found my way to a new, complementary modality of cancer treatment. I crossed into uncharted territory.

Every story is composed of many fragments like a kaleidoscope, and each fragment begs the question of what it means to be human when faced with the challenge of insurmountable odds. At times, the diagnosis of cancer reduces life to basic physical survival, which at times may appear mundane or even gruesome. However, paradoxically, these circumstances forced me to confront matters of the spirit. I observed the dedication of oncologists as well as the heroism of patients and their families who were required to wrestle with immense torment and physical constraints. All were compelled to confront their living and the inevitability of their deaths. During my hospital stays, I met with fellow patients with terminal metastatic cancer persisting in futile clinical trials in the hope of helping future generations. And the ones I spoke with only shook their heads and said, "It's just the right thing to do." However redemption is at the heart of any healing story and this is impossible without the transforming capacity of love. The fulcrum of healing is found in a balance between the disease and family. Viewed in this way, the physician is obliged to branch out beyond the individual patient to the wider network of the patient's closest allies. Therefore, cancer not only affects a singular life, but it also has the power to fracture and stress the very fabric of family, friends and colleagues.

Finally, in order to protect the identities of the people in this book, I have in most instances scrambled names and places with the exception of my personal family members. Since this book is drawn from my own experience in being healed from cancer, my encounters with qigong masters, oncologists and fellow patients are part of the fabric of my healing story. Readers should therefore use caution: This narrative is purely one individual's path towards cancer recovery. Therefore, I urge you to practice and follow the qigong exercises within this book only under the proper guidance of a competent and compassionate qigong master. Proceed with caution and in all cases, let your physicians serve as your primary guides and use the online network judiciously.

CHAPTER ONE: RUDE AWAKENING

By guiding a thin knife where there is ample space between the joints, one can carve up an ox without ever dulling one's blade. This is following the path of least resistance.

"You have lymphoma."

The oral surgeon pronounced apologetically after reading the summary of my PET Scan. In the silence that ensued after the bolt of lightning, I watched in slow motion as my wife, Janet, teetered, faltered and finally crumbled to the floor. How strange, at that moment, I couldn't feel anything.

"There is a great oncology team at the Weill-Cornell University hospital where I did my residency. They specialize in lymphoma. I highly recommend that you set up an appointment with them as soon as possible." As the surgeon spoke, I detected a slight tremor in his voice. Then, he handed me the folder with the scan, as if passing a football—aye, now it's up to me to carry it to the finish line, I thought. How strange that a routine tooth abscess shape-shifted into cancer. Now, the oral surgeon who performed the initial biopsy, having done his job handed me over to the oncology team.

With a sense of finality the receptionist at the front desk waved and wished us "Good luck" as we left the office. I felt a tightening of Janet's hand in mine. Yes, luck is what I sorely need at this point.

Later that day, Janet spoke to me with brutal honesty as she assessed our circumstances. "Well, we will just have to sell everything and make other adjustments; and if you are gone, I'll probably have to share the loft with roommates." I was enraged by the image of my wife in her middle age living with roommates, but this was the possible scenario in the event of my demise.

I gazed upon the abyss of my dark future, fraught with horror and suffering. As a father of three daughters with two of them still in college, I had to face the pitch-dark tunnel of a cancer diagnosis. I realized that I might become the dead weight that could strain and eventually tear the fragile fabric of my family both emotionally and financially. I imagined myself paddling in a small kayak with my family aboard, setting out into frigid waters filled with icebergs and ever-changing water canals. Being the chief of a minuscule tribe of five, I felt completely incompetent to care for them and I confronted the possibility that I might capsize our small vessel. I sat for a long time and in my mind's eye, saw beyond the event horizon: surgery, radiation and chemotherapy. Moreover, if these treatments should fail, then a bone marrow transplant would be the next course of action. Each path was filled with unendurable suffering and perhaps unimaginable disfigurement. Having no major medical insurance at that time except for hospitalization, the oral surgeon demonstrated genuine compassion in giving us a discount on bills and other services. In his eyes, I saw fear and concern. He recommended that I see an oncologist the very next day. Obviously, he was eager to pass me along to someone who had more expertise in the arena of fighting cancer.

As I assessed the path in front of me, I realized that I had no "good" options. I felt as if I was stuck in quicksand and with each struggle to free myself, I sank further down. I felt impotent, forlorn as if a mauling yawning jaw were closing down upon me. I had the sensation that a gigantic pair of insulation mittens were pressing the sides of my head, squeezing out every drop of hope. I hit bottom when the last breath of self-composure was knocked out of me, and in dark despair, I wept upon my wife's shoulder for the first time ever. I could feel her body bending and shivering slightly under my weight as she tried to fold me in her arms. "I am so awfully sorry to lean on you," I silently whispered. Then, I heard her reply, "In sickness and in health."

Unable to sleep, I spent hours on the Internet searching for alternative healing modalities—macrobiotic diet, vegetarianism, positive thinking— each one claimed to be effective in the fight against cancer. Completely overwhelmed, I turned off the computer and went into the front room of our loft and meditated. Gradually, strands of stillness began to gather and a distant, childlike voice sang to me. "Look into your roots, your own intuitive wisdom." This faint song revived me like a spring breeze easing my constricted heart and igniting a spark of healing power within me. Suddenly, a hope filled path emerged in front of me: Heal the whole person to cure the illness.

Cancer is not a sickness like an infection or a physical trauma such as a fractured bone. Cancer is a genetic disease with the contributing toxic factors such as aging, over-stress and an imbalanced organism, thus putting the whole organic system into chaos. After decades of stress my abused immune system had deteriorated and could no longer control the proliferation of tumor cells. A distant call to battle arose in me and the warrior awakened for the epic struggle between sickness and health, light and darkness, and ultimately, life and death.

A wave of sensation overwhelmed me, a sea-swell that heaved from underneath my chest buoying me up, and lifting me tenderly as if I were a small sea turtle thrown back from the sand where it had once been hatched. I had been returned from a world of raw exposed perils to my true element, the pull and push of tides. I became weightless, lightheaded with delicious hope.

The Crossing

One maple-crimson autumn, at a parents' weekend visiting my youngest daughter, Singha, the Maine air was already crisp and filled with the scent of musky fallen leaves. My wife and I had driven from New York City early in the morning and met up with her at the college dining hall.

"If you don't see an oncologist, I will not come back home…e-v-e-r," proclaimed my youngest with blazing eyes from across the dining table. I was shocked into silence. Checkmate. Since the initial diagnosis of lymphoma resulting from the biopsy, I had chosen to pursue an alternative healing route which included an intense course of dietary supplements, qigong, meditation, fasting and daily self-administered acupuncture treatments. I had lost almost thirty pounds and still, the tumor in my upper jaw (the maxilla) had continued to grow. From my perspective, being trained in Chinese Medicine as well as in qigong therapy, I firmly believed that I could manage and heal myself through these regimens alone.

Battling cancer was and still is a lonely journey, and I did not have a support system in this alternative healing modality. I prayed silently to the universe to send me a guide who had successfully traveled this path. I lived on a small island of daily struggles, practicing the qigong walk alone on the roof for hours and in public parks. In the early days of my sickness, I would stroll along the park lanes and assess its denizens' state of health applying my laser sharp gaze honed through many years of healing practice. Perhaps unconsciously I wanted to make sense of my predicament and to know why I had cancer and that old man, seated all crumpled with age, did not.

Being a healer and having cancer is a strange conundrum. Understandably, many of my students reacted with various degrees of fear, anger and help-lessness. Some even felt betrayed by their teacher, their master healer, how could he succumb to such a disease. After all, weren't the methods that I taught supposedly able to prevent cancer? Despite my best efforts to allevi-ate their fears and dissuade their anger, some departed and never looked back. Fortunately, a majority of my students remained with me.

Sometimes late at night, seated in deep meditation, I would feel utterly isolated and lost. The event horizon was enshrouded in darkness—a mo-rass of bleak unknowns. The myriad voices—the cacophonies of hawkers selling their own special brand of cancer cure became too bewildering. In this deep dark anguish, I cried out to the Bodhisattva Kuan Yin, "Oh, Bo-dhisattva, the all-encompassing compassionate one, hear me, please show me the way toward healing and send me an Earthly guide to lead me out of this jungle of despair." Somehow, I held firmly to the belief that if I had faith in the spontaneous healing power, I could cure myself.

My resolve was shattered by my daughter's threats. Finally, Jimei, my el-dest, beseeched me to see an oncologist. All three of them banded together in a united front and reluctantly, I acquiesced. Somehow, it seemed more selfless to do it for them then to do it for myself, but in hindsight, their demands saved my life. I shudder to think of the unbearable suffering that would have befallen my family had I persisted in my willful ways and not heeded the demands of my daughters.

"You would have been dead within a year," said Dr. G, my integrative on-cologist, unwaveringly. At my initial consultation, he told me that if I had kept to my original course of treatment, I would not have survived.

My poor wife would sometimes tease me that I would only listen to my daughters. My submission to their request and finally my return to health empowered my children giving them a sense of hope. Seen in this light, healing occurred not only for me, the individual, but also for my whole family. I had thought that I was isolated, but in truth, the guide was always present in the caring, loving voices that surrounded me.

As a result, I was able to find a way that would combine both Eastern and Western modalities of healing, and this book is a record of this passage. In my utter panic, I had wished for a guide who had already cured his/her cancer by these means. In some ways, my wish came true. With my cancer cured, my health restored; I can now serve as a guide and inspiration for others.

What is the Complementary Therapy Alternative (CHA) modality? Essentially, it is everything that I had been doing before the additional treatment of chemotherapy, which in my case was 12 cycles of R-chop chemotherapy. The process of Complementary Therapy works in conjunction with established Western medical treatments, helping to alleviate the negative side effects of these more invasive toxic means as well as facilitate the natural healing capacities of one's body, mind and spirit. It is a partnership that gives patients a better chance of fighting cancer.

After two months of attempting to exclusively treat my cancer with a detoxifying diet, herbs and qigong, it was evident that the tumors had continued to progress. However, stories of spontaneous healing by these means have been reported, but as of yet there is no scientific verification. Such rare occurrences are perhaps exaggerated and have become woven into the fabric of human belief. Facing a deadly and potentially fatal foe, I clung to these tales to give me hope. Fortunately, I was able to cross over to the CHA modality. I know this is a personal journey, but hopefully, my story can at a minimum serve as a stepping stone for others' healing quest.

Having trained in Traditional Chinese Medicine (TCM), I was able to slip into the CHA stream like a fish to water. Blessed to have these great weapons and the ability to harness them, all traces of the cancer were eradicated by the second round of 12 chemotherapy cycles without secondary effects (nausea, constipation, swelling, sores, weight loss). As an update, during my most recent checkup my oncologist told me that he relayed my experience of CHA to his patients and the possibility of bypassing all secondary side effects with acupuncture and qigong. However, my regular oncologist is not a fan of unproven dietary and herbal supplements.

In the past, the established medical treatment of cancer focused on the destruction, surgical removal and suppression of tumors and cancerous cells. This systemic shotgun approach induced great stress on the patient's physical and mental health. Subsequently, many cancer patients did not die from the disease itself, but from the treatments' side effects. Thankfully, as understanding of the disease and its cures progressed, scientists and oncologists would gain a much better understanding regarding the nature of cancer. Cancer is a vast category of diseases, encompassing a heterogeneous assortment of diverse types; even the field of lymphoma contains more than eighty different subcategories. Each cancer requires its own specific and individual plan of attack. At the frontier of this approach, new chemotherapeutic agents have been synthesized in labs to target specific cancer cells. These forms of designer drugs are less harmful to patients. However, only a few types of cancer respond well to these types of gene targeted treatments; a majority of late-stage cancers still have very poor survival rates. Hopefully, these shifting strategies will be able to address the fundamental issues of cancer treatment without debilitating effects on the patient's biological systems. This has been certainly true for me.

Since there was no well-established trail map that could guide me, I had to cull from a variety of different sources to create my own healing path. This book is the compilation of my personal field notes in my individual battle against cancer. May this book add to the vast arsenals to combat this overwhelming deadly nemesis.

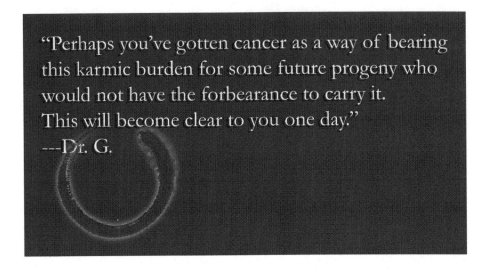

"Perhaps you've gotten cancer as a way of bearing this karmic burden for some future progeny who would not have the forbearance to carry it.
This will become clear to you one day."
---Dr. G.

CHAPTER TWO: O KARMA

How does one comprehend the whole story of healing from such illness? As in any story there is a beginning, a middle and end. Is the story concluded when one is cured? Or when one dies? How can the suffering, alienation and eventual triumph over this most insidious and deadly disease, be recounted to another?

As a young boy in China, I used to collect jellyfish. There are certain blue iridescent ones with glasslike tendrils that are so delicate they are almost impossible to capture whole and will break under the slightest touch. You must coax them gently into a porcelain bowl by letting them float and flutter on the seawater of their own free will and then scoop them up briskly into your receptacle. Perhaps this might be the way to relay these events—as completely as one can so as not to shatter its delicate, intricate life.

In a ground floor doctor's office located within a red-brick building covered in ivy, Dr. G walked in with his snow-white lab coat—a doctor's coat of armor and purity. His cheeks, mottled with pink, contrasted his deep brown iris which shone a penetrating gaze of both compassion and unflinching toughness. You have to be tough to be an oncologist, constantly battling against disease and death, a profession where victories are few and defeats overwhelming. Right away I knew that in facing this deadly foe, I could trust him.

"Hello, come on in," Dr. G spoke with a warm lilting Texas accent, the State where he grew up and went to school. "Would you like some tea?" he enquired.

"Yes," I answered and he left the office crossing the reception room to fetch us the tea. Janet and I were both astounded by this singular act of kindness and humility. It was the first time seeing a doctor that I was offered tea, and served in person by him. Only later would I discover that Dr. G does everything personally, from drawing blood to working his sound healing thumping instrument on my chest.

"I see from your scan that you have stage-two lymphoma. This type has a very good prognosis, and is curable." After handing us our tea, he settled in and leaned back slightly on his swivel chair. I sense—I can almost see—that at this juncture, Dr. G was mentally working through a series of clinical calibrations regarding the best approach to treat my cancer. Yes, this Chinese patient is a Traditional Chinese doctor, a qigong teacher of some renown—even one of my patients has studied with him. He has tried alternative healing with qigong and fasting for almost two months to eradicate the tumors, but it has failed and his face is swollen with the aggressive growth within the maxilla region, so that he has started to look almost simian. He is, Dr. G decided, a throwback to a feudalistic Chinese aristocrat, a scholar that needed the elegant argument of metaphor, Buddhist karma. I saw him arrive at his conclusion. I nodded in silent agreement.

"Normally, I would not tell my regular patients this perspective, but I know that you are a Buddhist and thus, well versed in the doctrine of Karma the continuity of action passing from one generation to another." Dr. G started his preamble in both acknowledging my culture and religious sensibility.

"This devastating sickness, cancer, might seem completely impossible to you, after all, you don't smoke or live in a radioactive environment. Many cancer patients have lived very healthy lives until the discovery of their cancer." Dr. G paused to take a sip of his green tea and allowed his words to sink in. "But you might one day suddenly recognize that what you have acquired is a karmic burden too heavy and overly strong for one of your progeny, a grandchild or great grandchild. You have taken on this karma because you have the strength to bear and cure it. Someday you will come across that individual, and he or she will spark a sudden recognition, and then you will say, 'Aha, that's the one.'" Dr. G explained this insight on our first consultation. As he started to speak, I felt a distinctive internal click of connection as I recognized the possible complement of alternative healing methods with standard western medical treatment. For me, Dr. G had become the bridge from West to East allowing me to cross over and accept Western medical treatment.

From the Buddhist perspective of karma, life is a never-ending story. You can envision it as a pebble being dropped into a cosmic pond with ever expanding ripples extending outward to the very end of time. So, in order to digest these momentous events it is very crucial that a framework be established to contain one's particular story of healing. For me, I conceived it as a perilous journey. My battle with cancer at the chemotherapy stage was like climbing a sheer, razor-sharp cliff demanding great consciousness, technology, and oh so many minute rituals comprised of chemo cycles, drinking water, measuring the output of urine and several other ceremonious routines. Yes, during this "cliff hanger phase" I perceived each ritual as a passage toward healing much like the small spirals a pilgrim walks within a sacred labyrinth. Every two hours one is woken up to check vitals, at early dawn blood drawing, then the daily sunny doctor's visit accompanied by the gaggle of white coated interns. This metaphor gave me a way to frame my chemotherapy treatment of 12 high-dose cycles scattered in cycles of 21 days—the magic number of cellular regeneration.

With the informative part of the consultation finished, I was led into the treatment room, and as I lay upon a soft leather recliner, I was serenaded by the soothing chant of Indian music. I had expected the standard procedures of blood pressure cuffs and heart monitors, but instead Dr. G asked me to lie down and close my eyes. Meanwhile, Janet settled on the other side of the room watching a most intimate rite of passage—the transmission of the heart. He turned the lights off and started to place a single elephant size headphone on my chest, and I could feel the deep infrasonic call of humpback whales singing in the deep sea and luring me into a somnambulistic trance. In the darkness, I returned to the primal womb of consciousness where I existed as pure vibration, with the thumping from the headphone resonating in my heart. Like a green sea-turtle swimming in the emerald silence of the ocean, for the first time since my sickness I felt that I was on my way home and a flicker of light beamed out: I will be cured.

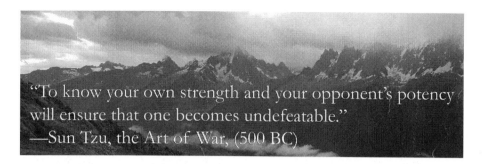

"To know your own strength and your opponent's potency will ensure that one becomes undefeatable."
—Sun Tzu, the Art of War, (500 BC)

KNOW THY ENEMY

The archipelago of human civilization is like the growth of coral reefs, tiny microbial crystalline organisms laying down their bodies as mortars for the next generation to build and develop a whole colony of coral into exotic aquatic boulders and flower-like forms of iridescent flaming colors. Metaphorically, our human civilization has followed a similar course as successive generations have been built on top of older structures as many mosques are built on top of Hindu temples. In an old Italian site, archeologists discovered beneath cellars of ancient houses, hidden remnants of a medieval town once sacked by a vengeful Catholic Pope, who had raged against the town's people who dared to stand against his will. He ordered his soldiers to completely obliterate the town forever by burying it out of sight and existence.

Yet, the unique characteristic of our human archipelago soars with the virtual imprint of the mind: our books, ideas, inventions, operas, arts, religion…All these we can pass down to the next generation.

Upon each successive layer of our human coral reef, cancer has been dodging us like a shadowy ninja assassin throughout the ages. During the Neolithic age, shaman excised tumors from the skulls of the afflicted by drilling holes with dull stone chisels. Many eons later, the Persian queen, Atossa, (550 BC) swaddled her cancerous deformed breast in cloth and then in a fit of raw primal rage, demanded a slave to lop it off like a rotten melon. As we leap forward to the present era, President Nixon declared an epic war on cancer on December 23, 1971. Over this vast expanse of time, victories against cancer have been few and defeats many. Cancer statistics have shown that in late-stage metastasized cancer only a meager 5% improvement in the survival rate has been evidenced despite billions of dollars pumped into cancer research and treatments.

Perhaps one needs to look at this disease called cancer in a new way. Rather than seeing cancer as an all-encompassing pathology—a singular disease, we should view it as a diverse population of heterogeneous diseases, which can be as varied as species of fish in the oceans. According to my oncologist lymphoma alone has close to eighty variants.

One must see clearly that cancer is our biological dark twin with its monomaniacal replication and survival tactics that take a lion's share of our life force. We must, therefore, track the evolutionary biography of this dark ninja. So let's retrace our steps from the present to the last fifty years to review how the battle between the two forces transpired.

FIFTY YEARS' WAR: ELUSIVE ADVANCES IN THE RACE TO CURE CANCER

Cancer, the final frontier of medicine has always been a high priority for modern medicine, for cancer knows no boundaries, age or race, and its occurrence seems to appear in a randomly chaotic fashion. Is it just bad luck that one is stricken with this most fatal disease? Since the war on cancer began, the National Cancer Institute has spent $105 billion in cancer research alone. Furthermore, other government agencies, universities, drug companies and philanthropies have added uncounted billions. The Susan G. Komen annual pink ribbon marathon has millions of women walking to support the fight against cancer. Nevertheless, in spite of the Herculean efforts and untold amounts of time, the death rate for cancer, adjusted for the size and age of the population, dropped only 5 percent from 1950 to 2005. (This statistic only applies to late-stage cancer with metastasis.) In comparison, the death rate for heart disease dropped 64 percent in that time, and for flu and pneumonia it fell 58 percent. After trillions of dollars invested over a span of fifty years, and with its success rate stagnated at only 5% total, if this were a publicly traded company, this would be extremely poor performance, indeed. Its CEO would have been probably fired in disgrace long ago.

However, due to propaganda, sleight of hand and a public feverishly wanting to believe in a cancer cure, the perception fed by marketers of the medical profession and pharmaceutical industry is that cancer is preventable with a certain diet. If that fails, it can usually be treated if the cancer is detected early enough, then it can be beaten with the ever new designer drugs. Regrettably, as many with incurable cancer have discovered, the picture is not always so rosy and the options few. And as for the early detection of breast and prostate cancer saving a life or extending survival time, there is no definitive clinical data to support such claims.

With all the efforts and money pouring into cancer research and the medical field, the dark ninja remains as potent and lethal as ever. Perhaps scientists and oncologists have been searching in the wrong place? Only if we can verify its true identity and nature could cancer be eradicated and possibly managed.

What is cancer—this dark ninja? The answer has always been intermingled within the origins of life on earth. The strands of DNA, which are mutable to the radiation from the sun, free floating radicals in our food and normal cell division, all give rise to mutation; in other words, evolution and cancer are the twin forces of life on earth—the yin and yang of growth and development of our species. There is, however, a major difference; evolution is organized life from natural selection, while cancer is primal chaos—anarchistic, a spattering of paint that spirals out of control. Life evolved from the blue algae of the deep primordial sea into ever more complex forms and inherent within this multiplicity is embedded the genesis of cancer. Hence, the hidden assassin is, in essence, our dark, evil twin who hangs onto life at all cost with fecundity in its self-reproduction.

We see now that cancer is not just an illness; it is a biological phenomenon. Cancer is akin to a multitude of invasive tentacles that drill and penetrate into the very core of our social, economic and scientific structures of society.

In other words, cancer exists as a microcosm within a larger world. It has all the components of a macro life form: self-organization, vascular growth and almost an uncanny survival instinct. Cancer is a perfect holographic reflection of our Earth in its present state of chaos. As we poison the Earth with our technological advances and industrial consumption of resources, the increase in the rate of cancer reflects the unhealthiness of our environment. In order to heal cancer, we will have to clean up our environment and reestablish the precious balance of life on Earth. This is the macro healing. It takes the whole Earth to heal cancer.

Warriors in the Battles Against Cancer

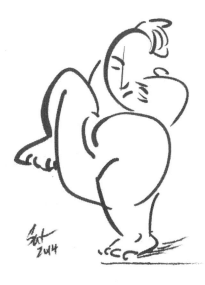

Dr. M, a tall man in his early thirties walks in. The first thing I noticed was the keen light in his eyes that seemed to look behind the façade of symptoms directly into the ephemeral realm of blood pathology. His pale blue eyes reflect the icy hue of the glacial lakes of his native Sweden. Being so tall, he hunches slightly to lessen his stature in order to make his patients feel less intimidated. He speaks with the precision of a scientist reflecting his background both as a researcher and clinician. He sat on the same side of the long conference table with us and proceeded like a mountain Sherpa to meticulously guide us through the minute steps of my cancer treatment's detailed plan.

"There are over 80 or more genetically diverse lymphoma, your type is called the large B-cell aggressive lymphoma which due to its hyperactive reproduction can be cured by chemotherapy. In contrast, the chronic, less aggressive type of lymphoma is not curable but can only be managed into remission and controlled by taking medication."

As I listened, where Dr. G, the integrative oncologist, had punctured a hole in the dark cubicle of despair and hopelessness, Dr. M, the Lymphoma specialist, began to widen the aperture into a stream of illumination. Mentally, everything clicked into place, and for the first time, I could see the whole path lying ahead of me—a steep climb clinging on a vertical jagged cliff face with the churning roiling waves crashing beneath. I would be climbing with a lifeline extended from my oncologists above with my life literally dependent on it. All my years of training in rock climbing, caving, meditation and qigong came into focus. They would be my tools, my pitons and spikes as I navigate the handholds, footholds and traverse the landscape of the ill.

Suddenly my body shuddered at the immensity of the challenge ahead, "What's it going to be like?" These were the unspoken words I never asked the doctors. And that'd be an obtuse sort of question, even if I could voice it. Not how is it going to be, but whether it will be to my liking or not. However, few say it out loud, so what could I do but brave the onslaught of the headwind and charge ahead. 'Damn the torpedoes, and full steam ahead!' from the battle cry of a long-forgotten sea captain.

The 12 cycles of highly toxic chemotherapy required at least 6 in hospital stays to monitor my body's tolerance of this poisonous cleanser—a brew of modern alchemy. And then I recalled what my climbing instructor had told me, don't look down and don't hug the cliff wall, keep your hands at shoulder level and don't over reach. Somehow, those directives became poignant strategy in my battle with cancer.

In any case nobody voices it aloud, so what can you do but ignore the smells and peruse the list of side effects (around sixty per drug) divided among three categories: common side effects, uncommon side effects, rare side effects. Death was unavoidably included, and was inevitably "rare," as in the example, "in some rare instances, death does occur."

A patient with cancer is akin to a traveler in a foreign country with its own sense of time, customs, etiquette and unfamiliar terrain. Time in this country of the sick is condensed into twenty-one day cycles (a common denominator for cellular regeneration). The process of chemotherapy has taken a cue from the agricultural practice of spraying insecticide to eradicate pests which in my case were the cancerous seeds (carcinomas). Each spray is precisely timed to kill off any new regeneration of cancerous growths which in my case were fecund. It is this particular distinction which allows my type of cancer to be cured. Large B cell aggressive lymphoma, with its invasive growth, can be killed off by repetitive chemo dosages. Dr. M had provided the gist of this insight of course in the dialect of a scientist conversant in cellular growth and cancerous stem cells. The analogy of pesticides comes from my own background in agrarian biology. Herein lies the paradox of cancer, the aggressive fast growing cells can be easily killed off and the sickness cured whereas the less aggressive, chronic kind of Lymphoma lingers within the system as cancer stem cells hide in the recesses of the body and await to relapse. These hidden cancerous cells might find their way into the brain, thus, as an assurance, six cycles of high dosage methotrexate—the first chemotherapy agent discovered in the 1950s—is prophylactically pumped into my brain to cleanse any roaming cancer seeds. The calculus of chemotherapy is thereby divided evenly between the lymphoma cells in the body and the roaming potential cancer seeds in the brain. The symmetry of this treatment became the gold standard for most lymphoma cancer protocols.

FIRST NIGHT ON THE ONCOLOGY FLOOR

On a windy October afternoon, two weeks after my initial consultation with the oncologist, I checked into the hospital for my first round of initial tests and chemotherapy.

It started to rain on the way over for my first night at the hospital. Riding in the cab, with Janet sitting next to me, I looked out the side window as droplets of rain fell in their own syncopated cadence on the glass forming strands of watery rivulets, canals and wiggling pathways that ran in different directions; their destiny mapped out. Strangely, it seemed to me that each droplet became a life trailing downward, sometimes, intersecting with others and enjoining into a single stream.

Since it was a scheduled hospital stay, my registration for admittance was smooth and without delay. The reception room in the hospital was uncharacteristically empty of patients unlike its emergency wing. Tugged away in the corner is the ever-present TV broadcasting old reruns of movie classics. By chance the channel was rebroadcasting *Lost*, a plane landed on an island with a group of survivors. How fitting as I was soon to be estranged on an island of my own, the 19th floor of the oncology ward. I would be for a week or so living with the denizens of the country of the sick, who carry their passports of the ill in the land of forlorn struggles, scans, and infusions of dark crimson liquid.

My room was a subdued pastel emerald green, a surprisingly vibrant color, with a painting of exotic floral blooms in a thin dark frame. My bed and section of the room were partitioned by a curtain that ran on overhanging railings which can encircle one's bed in a private isolated cocoon. The room perpetually gave off an astringent scent of pine along with the fetid odors of urine, vomit, bleach, and rubbing alcohol. All hung thickly in the air over something that was not quite stale, not too foul, but certainly not healthy. It was, I pondered, an odor of mortality. It was the scent of a place that had witnessed countless sufferings beyond human endurance.

Janet stepped gingerly toward the window and parted the thick heavy grey curtains. There below was the East River, an estuary, where the salty sea tide meets with the fresh water stream. Specks of pale white seagulls, and the occasional barge or sailboat drifted along in their slow motion grace. I had come to feel how time in the cancer ward slowed down, winding into a perpetual cycle of tests, pissing into the urine bottle, and the nightly insomnolent walks amidst the sounds of heart monitors and muffled coughs in the empty corridor. Across the river were stretches of small stores lining the bank. The streets were eerily deserted at this time of the night. Janet turned from the window, her eyes shining; she pulled a chair next to my vibrating bed and held my hand. I noticed how moist her palm was in mine. The room reverberated constantly with the beep of heart monitors as the silent drip of the IV kept time. Yet a pervasive gloom layered over this sonorous substratum of creaks, gurglings, and squeaks of rubber wheels on shiny linoleum.

I sat on the periodically vibrating bed and listened to the approaching footsteps from the hallway of the oncology ward with a great feverish sense of expectation, a visceral sensation so compelling and so vivid, so unfamiliar under any other circumstances that I decided then to simply name it after my native island, "Hong Kong". It's that Hong Kong feeling, and within it sprang shoots of hope and despair, anticipation, an almost hysterical giddiness of awaiting either the executioner or the savior, the good or the bad. I held an unvarnished faith as every time Dr. M materialized in his snowy white coat, he might, finally convey a test result so wonderful that the suspense of knowing its full extent or even its accurate assessment was overwhelming.

"May we sing for you?" A young couple shyly asked as they entered the room. No doubt volunteers from a church group, or maybe they have had a family member suffer the pain of loneliness in a fight against cancer, I thought.

"Yes, we would love to hear you sing." Janet replied, knowing how great an effort it must have been for these two young people, a tall slim man with dark-rimmed glasses carrying his electronic keyboard and a plump woman in her twenties still round with baby fat and a timid smile. For the first time in a long while, Janet and I both smiled. It was good to be serenaded by angels on my first night at the hospital.

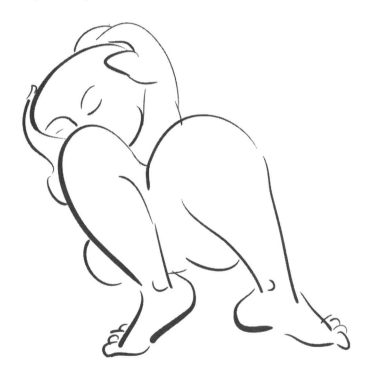

HEAVY METALICA

As part of the protocol of cancer treatment, a multitude of tests were given to assess my current state of health and rule out potential risks. The essential organs such as my heart and kidneys must be verified to see whether they could withstand the rigors of chemotherapy. Furthermore, it was necessary to see if any cancer lurked in the recesses of the body and brain. The oncologist is similar to a battle-worn lieutenant who sends scouts ahead to assess the terrain of the battlefield. He must also have a keen sense of his troop's strength and whether they can withstand the force of the enemy.

An echo cardiogram was taken to assess my heart's overall health and the technician told me that it was strong like a twenty-year-olds. A Pet-Scan will look for any hyper metabolic reactions of cancerous cells by injecting sugarcoated radioactive sweet water into the body. I was quite impressed the first time I was wheeled into the atomic lab for such testing. However, due to the blood-brain barrier, two other tests were given to assess whether cancerous cells had penetrated the brain: a spinal tap and an MRI scan of the brain. The spinal tap was done with a seven inch long hollow needle to penetrate the layers of skin, muscles and vertebra of the spinal canal and extract the cerebral spinal fluid (CSF). If the fluid is clear, this indicates that no cancerous cells have infiltrated the brain or spine. Of course, the CSF is examined in greater detail by a lab.

I endured all the other tests perfectly well with a quiet dignity and forbearance, a testament perhaps to my early martial arts training. However, the MRI scan turned out to be something quite unexpected. In the middle of the night, when the atomic lab is less busy, I was wheeled to the basement for my magnetic resonance brain scan. With quiet smooth efficiency, the lab technician slide me into the steel circular magnetic chamber, and my one-man shamanic trip began.

Here, right here in this cream white metallic sarcophagus, all my fear and courage, my illness is entombed. Here is my brain. Here is the convoluted grey matter that cognates with consciousness, pain and emotions. Here are the watery lights of my being—deep amber lights, purple-pulsating beams, shimmering, formless; lights that gather and scatter; here is the depths of my soul, the spirit within flesh; the unreachable essence that one dreams of, aches for, seeks after so frantically. Here it is, inside this steel chrysalis, in my deepest solitude. Without any warning, without the hint of its approach, I'm being bombarded by heavy-metal rock music, except that I am placed dead center on stage with this most thunderous Metalica band. I can feel my teeth chattering from the deep throbbing reverberation. Suddenly, I am filled to the brim of my being with overflowing love and joy.

Spontaneously without beckoning, a verse comes to mind, *I sing the body electric.*

DANCE WITH CHEMO

On a stark January morning, three months after my first consultation with the oncologist, I checked into the hospital for my second round of chemotherapy. The chemotherapy suite is a large, open space that included a reception room and treatment quarters. Seated in the reception area were patients waiting either for their consultation with their oncologists or waiting for their blood tests to come back in order to start their chemo. As I sat there by myself, a sense of calm and almost happiness washed over me. This is life that is common to all: the strong, the wealthy, the weak and the poor. Cancer does not discriminate. In this common bond, I felt something akin to elation and a sense of being part of a larger whole. As the Buddha proclaimed almost two thousand five hundred years ago, "Sickness is inevitable in life, as well as old age and death. The only option that exists is to liberate oneself from such suffering, therefore awake!"

O, Lord Buddha, I'm trying with all my might, I silently prayed.

After waiting 30 minutes in the reception room for my blood test, I was finally led to the chemotherapy suite. It is a small corner room that holds six or so patients receiving the intravenous drugs, some seated on recliners, others chatting on their mobile phones or listening to music with their iPods. I furtively glanced at my fellow patients. Most were wearing knitted caps from their loved ones or silk scarves to cover their bald heads. I noticed a young girl reclining on a brown sofa with her mother stroking her arm lovingly. Her skin was so pale and thin that the reddish chemical fluid being injected into her veins was clearly discernible. My heart ached for her and her mother. It was almost certain that the child was at the last stage of the chemotherapy cycle. As I strolled past her, the little girl gave me a thumbs-up sign to cheer me up. "It's not so bad after a few times." She smiled and spoke to me as I settled down next to her and began my own "al-chemo" drip.

Fortunately for me, the process of chemo treatment had been calibrated and titrated to the last drop. Initially, I was given a dose of antihistamine to prevent any unanticipated allergic reactions, which in the early phase of experimental treatment had caused a few deaths. Gradually, I started to drift over into a semi-trance state as my body absorbed the crimson fluid flowing into my veins. This particular formula of chemo described by the acronym of C.H.O.P. was comprised of four powerful drugs to cleanse my body of all traces of cancerous cells. Besides the four chemotherapeutic agents, I was given a cancer targeting drug, Retuxan, a chimeric monoclonal antibody which marks the cancerous B cells as well as normal B cells in order for my immune system to attack them later. Hence, Retuxan is not in the category of chemotherapy but rather a nontoxic cancer-targeting drug. The whole premise of chemotherapy treatment relies on the fact that the healthy immune cells are able to reproduce better than the cancerous ones. Even though the C.H.O.P wipes out most of the cancerous cells including the normal ones, the normal cells are healthier and can therefore regenerate better than the cancerous. However, chemo lowers the immune system to a very low level. With the addition of Retuxan, my oncologist explained that the possibility of curing my type of cancer was at 90%—a fantastic prognosis indeed.

In a large open room painted in a rather pleasant pastel shade of summer green, a half-dozen patients were already seated in their recliners. Pleasant bantering between the nurse and my neighbor seated next to me occurred like this, "How are you feeling this morning, Mr. X?" "I feel fantastic with the steroid. You know I have been trying to lose weight and now it occurs effortlessly." Ah, but there must be an easier way to lose weight, I silently reflected. As it turned out, the ambiance of the chemo infusion room was that of a Sunday buffet among strangers. We nodded pleasantly to each other without direct contact; each stayed within his bubble of solitude. It reminded me of the time I was in Japan's underground train station a few years back. Once the train arrived, professional packers gently pushed me into the carriage of a jam-packed train with their immaculate white gloves. Quite paradoxically, with my face literally inches away from the other passengers, my body pressed tight next to a diminutive salary-man, there was silence, solitude and anonymity, as if each was wrapped in his own temporary glass biosphere.

Chemo can be infused with a simple IV in the arm, or as in my neighbor's case, an implant of a small catheter port—a small silicone disc into the chest, which lead directly to the jugular vein. Due to its shape and the curved IV tube taped to the chest, it is sometime endearingly called a "piglet." In my case, my veins in my arm were able to withstand the corrosive effect of the chemo. I frequently felt a surge of adrenaline as the nurse pierced my arm with the needle, and the electric jolt never really vanished but dissolved into the effects of the steroid, the first of three bags of chemo liquid. The steroid calmed and modulated the peaks and valley of the other chemo drugs; I'd be charged up for twenty-four hours. As an aside, I discovered that steroids cause havoc with one's insulin level, therefore it is prudent to avoid any consumption of alcohol or sugary drinks within the 24-hour period, and even fruit juice is considered too sweet.

Once the infusion began, I would plug in my earbuds, turn on my iPad and watch a semi-documentary on the life of the Buddha. How appropriate it was to meditate upon the nature of suffering and freedom from it. For Prince Siddharta had given up his kingdom to find a path of liberation from the sufferings of birth, sickness, old age and death for all humanity. During the infusion, I watched the Buddha in his long enduring search for awakening. As the young Siddharta was seated in stone-cold meditation at the foothills of the Himalaya, I felt the icy chill of the blood-red fluid pump into my vein. The body sang its arias in slowly dissolving, cloud-shifting transformations, and a languor expressed in washes of flowing colors and the thick symphonic repetitive chord progressions of a Philip Glass opera. The form of these modulations was all swirling spirals—the organic geometry of nature at a cathartic tempo; the widening of the iris at the sight of neon blue electric eels in the deep sea kept pace with the chemo drips measuring time. All the while, the young Prince grew and became the Buddha attaining enlightenment under the Boddhi tree. In the final moment of awakening, the dark Lord, Maya, marshaled one last battle against the Buddha and hurled a thousand arrows, javelins, and flaming cannons towards the Buddha. With a single flick of his fingers, the World Honored One, the Buddha, transformed the slings and arrows into fragrant blossoms. So would I be able to transmute the poisons dripping into my body into medicine? The answer is a resounding YES!

One of the most inspiring core tools of healing is to have a vision that stretches beyond the boundary of one's cancer treatment. In this way, you are no longer pressed so tightly against the window of the cancer ward, looking longingly at the outside. Rather, you can see the possibility and hope of a life outside after successful completion of the cancer treatment.

For me, quite presciently, I had planned a workshop on qigong for healing cancer before the discovery of the lymphoma, and it was scheduled to take place two weeks after the last of my chemotherapy treatments. Lying in bed, with the IV of al-chemotherapy fluids dripping into my veins, I had a vision that I was hugging a young child with cancer and telling her that she will do fine as I had. In having such audacious visions, I become the captain of my destiny, and master of my own universe. I would no longer be a passive chaff buffeted by the winds of karma.

ABANDONING ALL HOPE

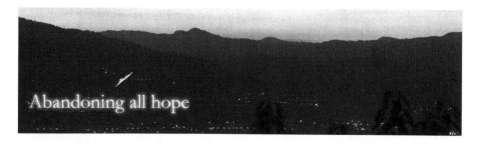

As the moon rises above the sentinels of water-towers, guardian of a million dreams.

Night deepened, a slight chill started to creep in as if from the dark clouds wrapping around the moon. I sat in deep meditation, Janet was sleepless in the bedroom. Bit by bit, holding the raw strands of darkening anguish, allowing the naked awareness to fill me, my consciousness crystallized into dark, obsidian—gradually an old repressed memory of my Taoist master bubbled up. He was seated with a group of his students in a restaurant. A middle-aged waiter with soft full lips and the glowing eyes like an owl's walked with springy steps and brought out steamy plates of dumplings. My master jumped up and greeted him like a long lost relative.

The proceeding conversation occurred in Chinese which I have taken the liberty to translate into English. "Chang, You old rascal you, how do you do?" Acting quite out of character, my master heartily pumped the waiter's hand. "Would you be so kind as to bestow words of wisdom upon my disciples?" he asked.

"Oh, your master is too kind. I'm but a lowly waiter with nothing to teach." The waiter demurred and bowed slightly in a way that reminded one of a ballerina curtsying to thunderous applause.

"Ah, no use in hiding now, you old sly fox. Just one lesson from you will benefit them for the rest of their lives." My master prodded.

"Well, if you've time to waste. Please continue eating while I entertain you with one of my tales." Chang went around the table and started to pour tea for each of us.

"This is the story of how I came to America. Lacking money for a fare, I bartered and worked as part of the crew on a tanker crossing the Pacific Ocean. It was the biggest ship that I had ever worked on. Nevertheless, when there was stormy weather, I could feel how it was tossed around by the waves like a toy boat. After we had been at sea for a fortnight, a typhoon started to develop in the middle of the night. The thickening storm concealed the world in pitch darkness and roaring waves. Occasionally, searing jolts of white hot lightening ripped through the darkness and sent sparks exploding the tanker's satellite dish. The captain sent the crew scuttling to tighten the cables and secure the cargo boxes. I wore a life jacket as a precaution, especially since I didn't know how to swim. As I lurched and teetered with each gigantic sea swell; it was so black on deck that I could see only small patches of light from my head lamp. On either side of the tanker, I saw a rising surge of glassy mountains with foaming white caps pressing toward the ship like giant hands clapping together as if catching a fly. Somehow, the tanker was able to just squeeze between them. We were tossed around the deck like match sticks." At that moment, the kitchen bell rang and Chang had to leave to bring out our other dishes.

After Chang returned with our dishes, none was in any mood to eat. We were mesmerized by his cliff hanger on the stormy sea. "Squalls of hail and bone-chilling avalanches of sea water penetrated every part of my body while an acrid bitter taste filled my eyes, ears and mouth. I fought to crawl up one of the cargo boxes to tie down the flaps with cables. As I stretched out to tighten one last loose cable, a sudden crash of ice cold swell breached the ship and swept me off my feet. I was swept overboard.

Immediately, the world vanished. Sounds, sights disappeared and suddenly a sharp freezing numbness choked me and instinctively forced my breathing to abruptly halt. It was probably a good thing, for I would have sucked in and swallowed mouthfuls of seawater into my lungs and drowned. As I surfaced, I was surrounded by rings of fluorescent amber lights flickering around me like halos. I felt my body being sucked downward into the valley of the colossal waves. I doubt that anyone had seen me thrown overboard. Being lost at sea in the middle of a typhoon, I realized that I was as good as dead. I felt this overwhelming emotion of dizzying terror that coiled around my heart and I saw myself akin to a tiny bottle thrown into a mass of swells. With this realization, my mind became completely still, and I abandoned all hope; I ceased my struggles and spontaneously caught a glimpse of my wife rocking and singing to her baby daughter while gently waving her round plantain fan to shoo away the buzzing mosquitoes. With one final gulp of salty air, I silently said my farewells, good-bye my loves, I'm so sorry to have to leave you... then suddenly; I felt an enormous force lifting me higher and higher toward the heavens, I could almost see the faint lights of the Big Dipper. *So this is how death is,* I thought. Quite unexpectedly, I felt a momentary weightlessness and suddenly, I was abruptly dropped back down on a hard surface, the ship-deck. Lying there wholly drained, it took me sometime before I tried to stand up, my knees buckled, and I fell face down onto my fellow workers who grabbed hold of me. Then I just blacked-out." Chang smiled demurely as he related his amazing adventure.

"Later on, my crew mates told me that they noticed an orange blob floating in between the waves. They were quite surprised to discover that it was me. 'You're a damned lucky son-of-a-gun,' they said as each patted and congratulated me. Was it luck or did my lack of struggle allow the same force that swept me overboard hurl me back onto the ship? Had I struggled would I have drifted away from this returning force? From that night on, I have lived each moment as if blessed with grace." With liquid silent dignity, Chang gathered our dishes and retreated back to the kitchen.

Chang's words stood the test of time and pierced through to the present: The force that sweeps you off can be the same that will put you back. If I can come to know intimately the source and circumstance that caused the cancer, then I can harness the identical forces into healing. The secret is in abandoning all hope and ceasing all struggle. Only then, did my heart become calm and a deep resounding equanimity sang out from the core of my being. In surrendering, I will be healed. I'll survive and pass through this perfect storm. This became my mantra during cancer treatment.

THE DARK SIDE OF CANCER

Fighting cancer forces one to peer into the belly of the beast. My cancer began with a simple observation—a lump on the roof of my mouth and possibly ends with an open creative solitude as I stand all alone in the eye of the maelstrom. From my vantage point, I watched how acquaintances, friends, students and patients were both repelled and drawn by this nearly fatal disease. Each was drawn to cancer's underbelly which is filled with the shadow of depression and suicidal panic. The herd instinct kills off the weak, the old and the sick, a reflection of the Hobbesian law of nature with its raw red tooth and bloody claw. Humans in the wild are untrustworthy corrupt beings, so each must protect his or her own just as beasts in the jungle do.

Privately, I suspected my clients and students were frightened by my sickness. One, in particular, felt devastated and betrayed. I visualize her eyes narrowing in a state of shock, her mouth opening in a slow motion scream. "How could you have gotten cancer? You're a healer after all!" Some left scattering off to seek better qigong masters and healthier healers. The dark side of cancer reveals this unbecoming, but all too human "herd instinct", therefore my only secure ally was my nuclear family. My wife and three daughters were still the only ones on board my small kayak as I navigated the eerie icy labyrinth within the vast desolate landscape. Every part of this terrain hides code for battle strategies, and the whole universe seems to be dropping signposts to guide one toward healing. Cancer becomes the impetus for the appearance of an entire maze of signs—faint dots illuminating patterns yet to be known.

My own story abounds in a sequence of revelations, generosity, betrayal, stark depression and exhilarating celebration of the human spirit. They came under the guise of my first bewildering night in the hospital, when the young Christian couple appeared to serenade us; my roommate, a cancer researcher, has the same type and stage of cancer as me; or the soft lullaby sung from a speaker phone to a small child in isolation. The list extends to a length beyond time and space. Cancer became a sort of kaleidoscope refracting the shards of colored glass that make up the human heart and mind, its strength and weakness, compassion and narcissism. Even so, remaining deep within the recess of this kaleidoscope, there is, in the end, a faith in the sublime radiance of love tingling above, beneath, through and around me.

The petit bursts of nausea had a diverse spectrum of tactile and kinesthetic shades as the days after chemo went by. My body expelled a particular condensed form of cathartic nausea, akin to a cuttlefish releasing a dark inkjet of fear. The entire phenomenon ultimately reached a crescendo in one final regurgitation: a gurgling throbbing burning sensation. It felt as if the corporeal entity of my being mounted one last heave to purge its cells of the toxicity; a searing pain started in the sacrum and surged in almost orgasmic contraction up to the spine and squirted out the top of the cranium, the yogi's Crown Chakra. Unbeknownst to me then and only later did I find out that my experience was akin to the rising of the Fire Serpent energy in Kundalini Yoga. Subsequently after this episode, I felt quite normal again, as I return from the supra-normal, spiritual heart-mind opening back to the ordinary state of day-to-day life. Perhaps, it was the poison of the chemo that propelled my body and mind to extend towards this pinnacle of Being, my consciousness therefore induced into a shamanic supra-sensitivity. During one especially agonizing episode, I could swear that I was seeing particles dancing in the air—the molecular structure of reality revealed. Hence, being pushed into the dark abyss of chemo, I re-emerged into the light soaked fabric of the universe.

And then, from this climax of agony and ecstasy, I lost a small piece of my mind as the sequence of chemo treatments gathered its momentum. Tilting me toward madness, I imagined that I was a wounded lion besieged by its mortal nemesis, a pack of hysterically barking laughing hyenas. Friends and acquaintances who wanted to visit me and give me their secret herbal cancer curing formulas: St. John's Wart, Kumbacha, extreme vegetarian diet, hunger diet... and several even promised to pay for consultations with faith healers, shamans and homeopaths. All this became a cacophony of voices and I had to shut them out. I had arrived at what my oncologist, Dr. G called, "Chemo Brain."

DAIRY OF A MAD MAN—A DREAM

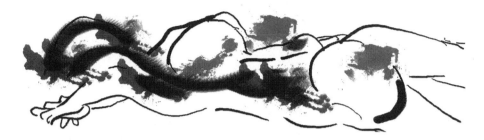

Drifting off to sleep, I felt my body splayed out until it covered the whole world; it became a shimmering thin transparent liquid film, stretching from one corner of the past to the present and even to the future. A disembodied voice resembling my late master's whispers, "All of time, past, present and future are already here in one complete whole. What has happened is still happening and what will come has already arrived and what is now will be alive forever." Forgetting that my body was splayed out, I tried to turn toward the sound and I felt the whole Earth turning with me. His words became a jumble of swirling concepts way beyond my comprehension. Through this film of time, gradually I perceived a lonely desolate, bone-dry wasteland extending for miles, and on this wasteland a massive upheaval of ant-like men fought each other in epic battles. The bone crunching sounds of feet stomped on little children, there was the wailing of bereaved mothers, toxic plumes of chemicals poisoned whole villages and row upon row of trenches filled with pale white corpses. Then from a distant rumbling, my body started to shake like a skin hand drum. There loomed on the horizon a fantastic mushroom shaped cloud that hyperventilated into the hollow breath of staggering death, I felt a burning intense heat melting my flesh and the ivory skull of death emerged from beneath, the radioactive clouds rained down on the people below. There were burnt crucifix structures everywhere and here and there were little mounds of dust, bones and ash all piled up. A small creature like a woodchuck sat on each mound in the desolate, cold, alien lunar landscape with bombed out craters. I wanted to shut my eyes but I couldn't, for this is the unblinking eye of time.

Finally after I woke up from this nightmare, my pillow was completely soaked through with a yellowish sweat. My body was extruding the chemo from its pores and I could almost feel ant-like itches running up and down my spine. Only later did I learn from Dr. M that vivid dreams are one of the side effects of chemo. How wonderful for me having never taken a single puff of weed or any other recreational drugs and now I am infused with a psychedelic liquid coursing through my veins.

DEATH, SURVIVOR AND WARRIOR

After a loved one dies from cancer, it is common for the family of the deceased to attribute the cause of death to something other than cancer: he died of cardiac arrest, or pneumonia, or massive organ failures...as if a death attributed to cancer would reveal something quite sinister and shameful. Cancer is menacing, not only as a contagion, like AIDS, but is an ostensibly, indiscernible tarnish to the very fabric of the individual's DNA. Surprisingly, with all the fund-raising events and cancer awareness media, this disease is still relegated to the underworld, not quite sinful or amoral such as AIDS had been misconceived upon its first appearance nevertheless, cancer certainly remains frightening. Cancer often infers a weak fiber of the individual's mettle. It is considered a blight, a curse, a divine wrath visited upon oneself, and henceforth the individual stricken with this disease must bear the burden and tough it out. By calling one who survives the ravages of cancer treatment "a survivor", we must recognize how we have been entrapped in this biblical undertow. In comparison, nobody in their right mind would accuse victims of a Tsunami, earthquakes or hurricanes to be lacking in character or mettle. However, in labeling individuals who manage to stay alive after cancer treatment as "survivors" we have unintentionally consigned the poor sods who died as pathetic failures. This is perchance the unspoken collective attitude of some families in their reluctance to attribute the cause of death of their loved ones to cancer. Let them die of a brain hemorrhage, kidney failure, respiratory difficulty but never cancer.

Comparably, when clinical data was published on genetic markers for certain cancers such as breast cancer, leukemia, melanoma, and ovarian cancer, this created sensational news. A cancer causing gene called an *oncogene* was discovered to be a hereditary factor that marked the individual person and their immediate family as "inferior". Women who possessed such a cancer-prone gene have chosen to have an elective hysterectomy and mastectomy before any onset of cancer. Those individuals with the oncogene are considered high-risk and their physicians would certainly suggest a vigilant regimen of annual scans and tests to catch the appearance of cancer as early as possible. This scanning and testing mania is based on the unproven premise that if cancer is caught early enough then the possibility of successful treatment will be increased. But it is not quite true. It is a false bias. To illustrate this case lets imagine identical twin sisters living in the same environment and community, one of the twins, Alice religiously had regular mammography and in one of the scans cancerous growth was discovered. Under the advice of her oncologist she chose to have an elective breast lymphadenectomy and chemotherapy but after three years her cancer relapsed and this time all standard treatments were unsuccessful in controlling the cancer, and Alice died five years after the onset of the cancer at the age of sixty-two. Now, her twin sister, Julie, did not have regular mammography and then one morning, she discovered a lump in her breast; the cancer had metastasized to the bone. After mastectomy and a bone marrow transplant, the cancer still relapsed, and she died at age sixty-two. Hence, this case illustrates the false bias of early detection in breast cancer. Unfortunately, this is not a fictional scenario but an actually clinical case study. In his monumental work, *The Emperor of All Maladies: A Biography of Cancer* by Siddhartha Mukherjee, an Indian-born American physician and oncologist, he cited this particular clinical case. However, a handful of cancers such as cervical and colon do benefit from early detection. On the other hand, the controversy surrounding early testing of a PSA marker for prostate cancer has proven to be without merit. The president of the Prostate Cancer Society himself vehemently refused to be tested for such a marker, his reason is based on the science that having such a test would not necessarily improve one's survival or extend the life-span of a patient but would often lead in most cases to unnecessary surgical or radiation treatment. Thus, to apply a general overarching policy of scans and early detection tests on the vast range of genetically mutated diseases is akin to killing a few fleas with a sledgehammer.

From the darkside of cancer, I have not only survived the cycles of chemotherapy, but I am now cancer free and cured. My health now restored, I personally do not feel like a passive survivor of a divine wrath. I feel empowered and victorious as if I have won a most decisive battle against this exceedingly lethal, odious shape-shifting foe. The only name I would call someone who has gone through such a battle would be a cancer warrior, a fighter for all that is life-affirming. Suddenly, unexpectedly a surreal image comes to mind: me kneeling down on one knee with sword drawn extended to you, the reader. It is my pledge and my honor to serve you in your fight against cancer. Everything that I have gleaned from my battle I offer to you. My experiment in Complementary Therapy is for your own healing and redemption. This is my vow.

THE WAVES OF SERENDIPITY

By surrendering completely without struggle, you allow the waves of serendipity to propel you toward your healing path.

Serendipity is the crisscrossing of events—a tangle of interwoven convergences. In my case, both my oral surgeon who discovered the lymphoma and my integrative oncologist, Dr. G pointed to New York Presbyterian Hospital for treatment, as it has one of the best hematology and oncology departments in the world. Kings and royalty of all kinds reserve whole floors for their cancer treatment.

Serendipity sometimes appears under the guise of an accidental stroke of luck when one stumbles upon something helpful without looking for it. In search of a holistic oncologist, Janet's colleague found Dr. G when her husband fell ill years ago. However, being raised in a conservative family, her husband had decided against seeing an integrative oncologist, as Dr. G's medical philosophy was too radical for his conventional sensibility. Quite tragically, he died when his cancer relapsed. Recently, his wife asked me whether I thought Dr. G's integrative treatment would have extended his life. "I don't really know," I replied. "It's hard to assess the potential outcome of an alternative approach. Nevertheless, based on my own experience, the complementary modality could have possibly extended his life."

Serendipity is a glowing message scribbled in the realm of chance encounters, possibilities and probabilities. For me, it appeared as a joint frontal attack by my daughters who threatened not to come home from college if I did not seek traditional treatment or a door suddenly swinging open on a cool autumn day caused a written note from Janet's co-worker to flutter down to the floor like a solitary lunar moth with the name and telephone number of Dr. G.

Serendipity is lying on Dr. G's exam table while he administered the deep, full-throttle chant of a Sanskrit mantra from his Guru into my heart. I felt the glow of an amethyst on translucent skin, and my pupil widened in semidarkness as I saw shimmering life enter my body—a jolt of transmission received, indeed.

Serendipity is how twelve years ago I had studied with one of the few qigong masters who taught the qigong walk for healing cancer, not knowing that one day I would be my own cancer patient to apply this healing technique in curing my cancer.

Serendipity is how only recently scientists discovered a special cancer targeting drug for my type of curable Large B-cell Lymphoma.

I have come then to see these harmonic lines of synchronistic events, people, and forces converging into a symphonic mantra—a raga of healing. A roaring crescendo orchestrated to eviscerate the cancer from my body.

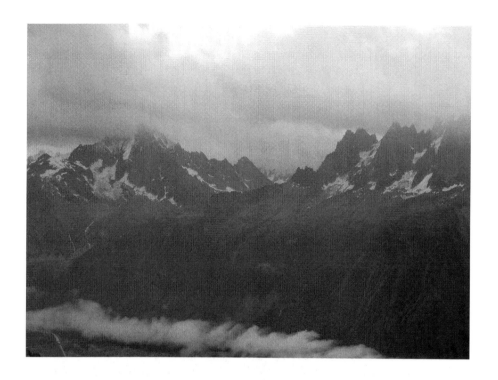

CHAPTER THREE:
THE BATTLE GROUND

Fighting cancer sometimes requires you to have the speed of a panther, the endurance of an elephant and the patience of a saint.

Having been trained in the art of meditation, I am nothing if not accommodating. I could remain utterly stone still as I was transported hither and thither between glinting giant doughnuts with their particle emissions, the cutting-edge wonder of modern technology infiltrating into all the nooks and crannies of my body. *Raise your arms over your head. Try not to move too much. Don't eat anything after midnight before the morning scan. Inhale and hold your breath.* These were the common refrains of the technicians. After thirty minutes in the metallic cocoon, I was spit out and whisked away to another room, for yet another test.

Different hospital departments conferred with each other regarding my results leaving me with nothing but a vague sense of foreboding, mysterious bruising, weeks of unimaginable fatigue, and plenty of time for my imagination to run wild or (heaven forbid) trawl the Internet to entertain my excessively active brain! The days leading up to Dr. M's consensus based on my bone marrow results and blood tests were the most unnerving. It was like being part of a battalion with feet shuffling on the chilly battlefield waiting for the moment when the commander points his sword and yells, "CHARGE!"

'It is possible to die,' I reflect briefly. *'I, or anyone, could react to chemotherapy.'* The treatment is full of potential deadly side effects: kidney failure, heart failure, extremely diminished white blood count resulting in immune deficiency. I needed to stay in the hospital to titrate the toxic high dosage of methotrexate which killed the cancerous cells by pushing one's body to the brink of death. After twenty-four hours, the nurse would swoop in to administer the rescue remedy of leucovorin, a strong dose of vitamin to resuscitate my blood, and then flush the toxin out of my system with bags of saline solution. The first time I felt the cold sharp fluid enter my veins, I shivered and my whole body started to tremble like a horse rearing at the howls of wolves. I reclined back into a deep reverie and recalled majestic peaks amidst a sea of swirling, curling mist.

My cancer treatment began with tests: PET scan, bone-marrow biopsy, MRI—that magnetic cocoon blaring thundering heavy-metal music directly into my brain, blood tests—the snapshot of overall health in daily, hourly sequences. In between were the rounds of chemotherapy infusions, the hospital stays to oversee the effects and flush out the toxins. Then finally in reaching the end of the chemo cycles, if the results reveal no sign of cancer anywhere the testing and observation phase resumes anew.

I felt that all the parts of the landscape including the vibrating bed, the jugs of urine hanging at the end of the bed, the windows facing the East River and the movements of the nurses with their bags of potent toxic drugs injected in my veins were a complex choreography. The dance of the whole microbial universe converged at the still point—the complete eradication of the cancerous cells from my body. Life at the hospital was a maze of faint dots of light swimming in twilight consciousness between IV drips, and my strolls—walking laps in a circular path around the oncology ward. Folded deep into the fabric of this dance, there is, ultimately, a faith in the extraordinary light of life surrounding and embracing me. I had a strong intuitive image that all I needed was to simply sit tight and let the river of life carry me over the rapids and boulders; that I did indeed.

There he is. I hear the thoughts of the night nurse as I stroll past while she monitors banks of computer screens at her station. The enigmatic, surprisingly serene Asiatic man with his shaved, round head and silk scarf wrapping his shoulders, out on his regular walk while the metal pole carrying his IV tubes and dangling bag of saline solution swing in time to his waltz-like movement. He has informed me that his lumbering strolls are a form of healing walk, Qigong. The way he walks has a certain gracefulness, a kind of animalistic charm and yet, tonight, he makes a heart-wrenching sight—teetering in his rumpled hospital gown and paper slippers, fighting the strain of chemotherapy.

Taking a rest between efforts, he stands like an old water buffalo already up to its knees in quicksand, massive and proud pretending to contemplate the tender grass on the far bank when it is startling clear that it will remain here, trapped and alone after dark, when the wolves come out. Yet, he perseveres with his walk, his warrior dance. He must have been an exquisite dancer twenty years ago; women must have fainted in his embrace. The night nurse is proud of her ability to dissect the history of a face; to recognize those who are now sick were once healthy. The light blinks for room 362 and she ambles off.

In the morning, my oncologist made his teaching rounds with his entourage of interns.

"Not interesting." These were the two words uttered by my oncologist regarding my PET scan after only two rounds of chemotherapy. "There is no trace of cancer cells anywhere!" I was giddy with disbelief. His two words, "not interesting" were magnificent. Could it have been that after a 21-day cleansing diet consisting of a single bowl of bone soup a day, my daily qigong walk and hours of deep meditation my cancer cell count had been reduced to a single digit of 6 or 7 even before my treatment began? In comparison, my roommate still had a cancer count of 67, even though he also had stage-two lymphoma and a similar type of cancer. Fortunately, after completing twelve cycles of chemotherapy, my roommate was able to vanquish all the cancer from his body.

"Maybe you didn't have too much cancer to begin with?" Dr. M. noted. A few months later, when I sent the early PET scan results, Dr. G rejoiced. "This is an excellent indication that you responded extremely well to chemotherapy," he told me. Both oncologists were unanimously agreed that my recovery "made their day". Subsequently, even with these fantastic results, Dr. M suggested that the rest of the chemotherapy treatments be given as a form of assurance.

Life from then on became a syncopated rhythm of 28-day cycles recovering from outpatient chemotherapy and interspersed with the deep brain infusions of Methotrexate—its toxicity being the main reason for my hospital stays. If my blood's acidity level became too elevated, the drug would form small crystal-like snowflakes which would act like tiny razors and cut my organs to bits. The nurse took a drop of blood and assessed the pH every twenty minutes or so after the initial infusion. I stayed in the hospital so frequently that when I returned home for short periods of 14 days or so, the very nature of time shifted; it seemed like an eternity. On the last day of my chemotherapy, the nurses brought out a small cup cake with a little birthday candle to celebrate the end of my treatment. Celebrate we did; I was born anew!

"Live your life," the oncologist on rotation advised me after my last chemotherapy treatment was complete. "Now, we just observe," she concluded. Life, having been snatched back from the jaws of death, covered everything with a verdant sweetness. Shortly thereafter, in a qigong seminar that I lead, someone asked me, "What is the meaning of life?" I responded "Life." The word tumbled out without any doubt, prefabrication or intellectualizing. That simple.

.

CHAPTER FOUR:
GLIMPSE FROM THE WARD

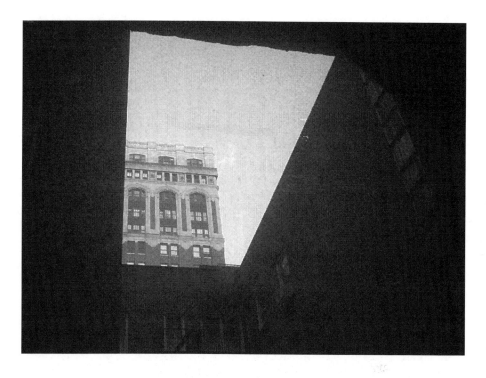

Being confronted with inconceivable suffering, our eyes appear wide open, but remain firmly shut. Perhaps, this arises out of the reflex of self-protection, a response to the launching of harmful projectiles both physical as well as mental.

NIGHT AT THE ER

On a taxi ride to the hospital, waiting at a red light, I looked out at the stream of people rushing headlong into their daily chores. Mothers walked briskly to pick up their children who fidget impatiently at the schoolyard, a middle-aged Chinese delivery man careened dangerously close to the traffic on his bicycle with bags of steamy General Zhao's Chicken dangling on the handlebars like crumpled paper lanterns, and then I saw my own reflection superimposed on the glass. I still looked all right; thin now instead of a physique composed of one too many midnight snacks. When will the gauntness, the baldness, yellowing fingernails, and cracked lips of my embattled face begin to fade? Outside, it started to rain and streaks of water formed on the windshield. The driver shouted a word in Panjabi and then the light turned green; the cab moved on. Seated next to me, I noticed Janet dozing off. Poor thing, she had hardly slept a full night since the discovery of my cancer. At that moment, I wanted to cradle her in my arms once more like the time she awoke from a coma after the difficult birth of our youngest daughter. I know she adores me and in a moment of revelation, she whispered that she might not continue if I didn't. I wanted to scream at her: You must live for the sake of our children. I grew weary of being treated like an invalid simply because my immune cells were bleached away by the chemotherapy. But now, a simple infection wrecks havoc on my body, sending my temperature to 103. And when I called the doctor's office, the phone message was clear: *If you have a temperature above 101, hang up and dial 911 or go directly to the emergency ward.* Then I discovered that Janet was not dozing, but crying silently into her hands. I believe—I know—that I would come through this tribulation and emerge victorious, and this was just one more wrinkle in the fabric of my healing story.

It was rush hour. The sky seemed to grow more ominous with the rain and distant sound of thunder. The lights from the buildings and cars turned into an impressionist painting of dots and dabs of color, blinking red and green. I recollected reading a pamphlet published by the Lymphoma Society that a side effect of chemotherapeutic medication was "a shift in vision." Everything appeared somewhat crumpled, as if the life force had been sucked out and suddenly I realized I was seeing double. Superimposed one upon the other were two-color plates of green and red, as if different colored inks from a printer were not registering. The city took on the appearance of a 3D movie except that I was not wearing 3D glasses. Either I was tripping on the massive dose of the steroid, Prednisone, or my brain was being fried by the fever. Suddenly, I felt Janet squeeze my hand. *You will be okay, just hang tight* a small voice spoke inside my head. *Ah, now I'm hearing voices* was the last thought before I blacked out.

An eerie tingling sensation, similar to the crinkle of tin foil seemed to wrap around my senses. A dull underwater sound boomed in the back of my brain. Wholly disoriented, I found myself floating in a sea swell back to the seashore of my native island, Hui Nang—as if I had been delivered from a world of raw unmitigated danger to my native tropical sea. I felt a gentle pull and push of the tide, that floaty, woozy mildly metallic oblivion.

As I slowly blinked, stereoscopic flashes of light and images filled my consciousness; I heard the distinctive sound of beeps. I woke up in a wing of the emergency ward with a private room—a privilege awarded to my immune deficiency. The beeps of the monitor registered my heart. My body was hooked up to various tubes, electrical wires and an IV. The nurse arrived and injected potent antibiotics directly into my vein. It was as if a unit of the Special Forces dropped down from helicopters into a barren landscape to destroy invaders. I could almost feel the ice-cold fluid coursing through my veins soothing my feverish body, saving me from the edge of a burning pit. Seated in a corner across the room, Janet was entangled in a small metal folding chair watching me intently as I regained consciousness. I tried to smile, but my lips were stuck together. Instead, I gave her a thumbs-up sign. I had survived the right hook of cancer and the left hook of chemo.

Outside in the ER corridor, beds were parked like ring of wagons under attack and filled with patients suffering from various traumas. All nightlong an old woman continually asked when she could go home; her husband patiently repeated, "You fell, you can't go home." "I want to go home." "You can't. You just had a fall." "I want to go home..." and then out of my peripheral vision, I see an orderly hurriedly wheeling a young woman out of the ER. "They decided to place her in a hospice program," whispered a junior intern to another.

"You are experimenting on me."

A young resident lingers a moment behind the others, giving herself a view of my old Jewish roommate's gaunt frail back with a spider web of tubes attached to his arm with tattooed with numbers. She is nearly panic-stricken by something other than what she currently perceives, but a deeper, more nightmarish image of Auschwitz survivors in a concentration camp. Earlier, while she examined him, she heard him mutter, "You're experimenting on me." Oh, how true, but it is for an entirely different end, she thought. She hastened to join her colleagues to make their morning rounds.

After the interns left, the old man's wife who had been seated stone-still slowly rose and went over to gently smoothing the few strands of grey hair on his forehead. Being so close to him allowed her a whiff of an assortment of his humors. His skin exuded not only his usual perspiration which had always reminded her of the faint fermented odor of the ancient wine cellar where she hid from the Nazis, but his blood-red medicine gave him a slightly tangy, caustic, acrid odor. He smelled, too, of unwashed laundry, although she had just changed his pajamas in the early-morning hours. More terrifyingly, it was the real nightmarish aroma of death—a rancid, putrid odor emanating from the vibrating bed he had been strapped into at night that caused her the most distress. His hospital bed was dying; the bed had accumulated so many deaths over the years, a multitude of heart-wrenching spasms and last great gasps of breath that it was difficult to detect whether he was living or dying. The bed, an oblong electric mattress balanced on steel rollers was restless; it shuddered with nervous energy. As it folded half way to prop-up the patient, it groaned into a seated position.

DANCING WITH MR. PING

At my previous chemo treatment, my roommate was a petite Chinese man wearing cotton pajamas printed with a thousand cranes all over them. His head, usually clean shaven, resembling ancient polished river-stones, but lumpy from tumors. His back bent after decades of washing mountains of stranger's dirty laundry, shoulders hunched in a perpetual apology with his arms hanging apathetically at his sides. He seemed less like a person and more like a sack of rumpled old clothes ready for the recycle bin. To most people that knew him, Ping was a man so seemingly simple that only a profound man would recognize the depth of the very simplicity of his Being.

Since his English was quite rudimentary with only a smattering of essential phrases (starch or no starch, ready by tomorrow quick, cash only), I volunteered to be his interpreter. But here is the rub, since Ping spoke only a wild village Fukien dialect with little resemblance to the common tongue of Mandarin, I therefore had to extrapolate his messages. It was, as is said in a Chinese proverb, a conversation between a rooster and a duck.

"Mr. Ping, Mr. Ping, wake up, time for your medicine." Victor, the night nurse, gently nudged him from his dream. Ping dreamed of luscious green fields of watery rice paddies with their oblong rows carved out of ancient cliffs, resembling steps for giants. The noon sun was shining little diamonds on those shimmering steps. Earlier in the night, before the night nurse's shift had begun, Ping cried out in agony caused by an impacted molar drilling bolts of lightning into his brain. The nurse didn't speak Chinese and it would have taken too long for the hospital's Chinese translator to arrive.

So I yelled out from my bed, "His tooth is killing him. He wants more morphine."

Sometimes during the rare silences of nighttime, I would overhear Ping singing soft lullabies to his little daughter on his cell phone lulling her to sleep, "Rowing and rowing to grandma's bridge, grandma has a little treasure child, a little treasure..." Without fail, I would fall deeply asleep as well. The magic of his calming voice was so hypnotic even the nurse would start to sway to the rhythm of his song.

In my profound gratitude for his soothing songs, on my last victory lap waltzing around the corridor with the qigong walk, I invited Ping to join me. However, before he decided to take part in this dance, the only question he asked was "Where did you learn this?"

"From the Buddha," I answered without missing a beat. With Ping waltzing behind me, outside fluffy flurries of snow swirled and hovered in languorous descent, only then, did I suddenly realize the heart of healing:

Breathing in, and breathing out, stepping right and stepping left, with Mr. Ping following behind me and white blossoms falling from heaven. That simple.

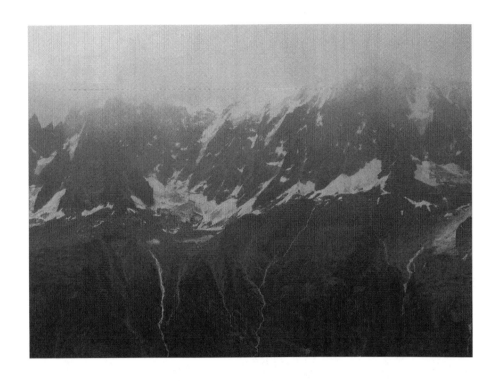

CHAPTER FIVE: THE MIRACLE OF QI

Deciphering, trudging into the nether regions, tunneling one's way through the macabre atlas of alchemy, startling darkness, unfamiliar flora and fauna.

Qi, is breath, emotions, vapor, weather, energy, and finally the fabric of the whole universe. The origins of Sino-linguistic words can be traced back to imagery carved on oracle bones from the Neolithic period. The most well-known and still widely used prehistoric oracle bone scripts are the eight trigrams of the I Ching, The Book of Change (10,000 BC). Each trigram consists of either single unbroken horizontal lines, — or broken lines, – – .

The South Korean flag incorporates the trigrams as symbols of power and antiquity. The four trigrams represent the sky and earth, sun and moon. Similarly, the word, 气/Qi (breath) captures the primal image of vaporous wispy fingers rising out of the glacial era or the Ice Age. Hence, each Chinese character is an icon that points directly to the reality behind the word. Chinese written characters have a direct visceral power that grasps one by the hair; as a young boy, growing up in China, I was literally afraid of the word "tiger."

Sometimes, there are concepts embedded in a specificity of a language that are impossible to translate into another. However, simply by examining the image of Qi as a visual symbol, its primary meaning related to the ideas of energy and breath starts to emerge. Death, accordingly, is one without Qi and someone who is extremely weak has depleted Qi. Qi permeates every stratum of life. The air we breathe is called Qi, the weather is called heavenly Qi, the outburst of emotion is called Spleen Qi, a tasty meal is considered to have good Wok Qi. In the words of one Princeton East Asian studies professor, "Qi is so damn common, you find it here and you find it there and you find it everywhere." (No doubt he had taken the liberty of paraphrasing his favorite film, *The Scarlet Pimpernel*.) I have tried in the following paragraphs to trace the myriad footprints of Qi.

Qi is a mesh of dark matter uniting, stretching and spanning galaxies; a nothingness beyond measure; a vaporized mist arising from rain forests on a summer's dawn; a baby's first gasp of air inflating her virgin lungs; the minute signals shared between organs.

How pervasive is Qi? A spark of consciousness descends and transforms into Qi; while a single drop of blood carries its essence. It is finer than the finest matter.

Qi is a sublime force emitted from healers to the ill; it can tease out dark pathogens and lance cancerous tumors out of their crustacean shells. It's the shimmering halo dancing on translucent skin; a sliver of ecstasy suspended beyond time and space. It is the conduit between consciousness and matter: an impulse, a widening pupil at moonrise, the glint of salmon-pink radiance at dawn; a subtle imperceptible motion of consciousness appearing at the leeward side of dream—a twilight state. It's the alchemical stream's reverse flow from matter to spirit, from fluid to vaporous energy and finally into light; the first breath; the spark of life.

All the world is but a gathering and dispersal of Qi—the cosmic breath. The tendrils of Qi reach out and penetrate all of manifestation, from the Crab Nebula to the molecular bonds of DNA.

What is Qi? It is everything and nothing; grasp and ye shall feel it escape through your fingers. Energy, breath, air, bioelectricity, gravity, emotion, force, weather…

WHAT IS QIGONG?

I hesitate to respond, as the answer to the question is not easy to formulate. Nevertheless, in my view, a simple and direct reply might be that qigong is a means to reconnect to the root of ourselves hence granting us access to a realm rarely perceived. Of course, as soon as the qigong practitioner puts his toes on the path, the more he recognizes that this connection comes at a price. One begins at first by attempting to decipher the macabre atlas of alchemy, tunneling one's way into a dark and unknown nether region filled with unfamiliar flora and fauna. Should one persist with such a conquering spirit into this unfathomable realm? With quivering senses one reaches out blindly in total darkness; a leap of faith is required to verify qigong's very existence let alone its healing power. However, now and then, a sumptuous vista will suddenly emerge, a slice of nirvana with gleaming limpid deep sea-creatures lurking in the depths just beyond the reach of our ordinary consciousness.

To begin this sojourn, we must first devise its Neolithic roots and oral history. In my case, I stumbled upon the practice of Qigong quite accidentally, or by fate (depending on how one views the events of one's life). I had expected to find the shuddering magic of sorcerers and alchemists, the stuff of myths, with shaman wearing iridescent cloaks and beatific sun-bleached skulls mightily beating seal skin drums. But in truth, it was something more akin to falling in love, the haunting revelation of a native son's home coming.

The dawn of Qigong arose at the origins of our common ancestry during the Ice Age with the mythic shaman Pan Gu, the Old Man. In this Chinese legend of genesis, Pan Gu cleaved the undifferentiated chaos or void in two, releasing light and shadow, thus sparking the birth of our universe into a dynamic interplay of Yin and Yang. The interaction of these polarities (complementary opposites) is the essence of qigong cultivation. Encircled by flickering glowing embers, the Neolithic shaman dances in the play of shadows with his feet dragging along the earth; this slow lumbering gait suddenly turns into a bear emerging from a long winter's night. The shaman is transfigured into part animal and part man.

In a simple lifting of an arm like a heron's pale ghostly wing, I was plunged abruptly into a luminous and mobile liquid that was none other than the pristine element of time. One shares it—just as excited archeologists share their rare finds—with ancient alchemists in their discipline of transmogrification.

Following the ancient's trail, qigong starts, not in the physical, but in the metaphysical plane where metamorphosis is a reality. One practices this archaic yoga to be transformed from a lowly leaf grubbing caterpillar to a full-fledged monarch with dark-eyed wings, freed from a humdrum existence in low lying shrubs. One drinks the honey, the dew of life and sheds the skin of mortality.

But how precisely did I end up in the field of qigong?

To start with, I met my qigong master after having trained eight-years in Taiji and martial arts. I was on the brink of liftoff into adulthood, perched upon my senior year at Princeton majoring in the field of neuroscience— otherwise known as, "the rat psychologists." Our subjects were mostly rodents in their primal urges of sex, feeding and aggression. I will spare you the details of my change in major from psychology to dance and my final professional fate teaching qigong. But, this much I should say: I grew up in communist China and was branded a landlord's son. It was an age still caught in the dying grasp of a feudal giant—"a rotting and putrid corpse," as Mao so succinctly put it—the collapse of 10,000 years of monarchy.

"Once upon a time in China, and such a very different time it was," became the oft-heard refrain of my childhood. Our family had lost everything: my father's import/export business and our two-story brick house overcrowded with destitute squatters who paid token rent with hungry mouths to feed. While my father and eldest brother were imprisoned in labor reform camp, my mother took the young ones and fled to Hong Kong. I remember holding my mother's hand as we stepped gingerly along planks of wood laid over unfinished steel beams of a bridge that spanned the border of China and Hong Kong—at that time, it was still a British colony. At this crossing, I could see the turbid muddy water rushing below the gaps in the planks.

I tried to wiggle my hand free from her iron grip but it suddenly tightened and squeezed the blood from my fingers. My vision became blurred with tears, as my mother with pale silence dragged me across the steel bridge. This was my rite of passage, my very first immigration into a foreign land.

We'd been lucky to adapt, but a world had ended. The end had come five years before my birth. And although I can tell you that I am neither a religious, nor superstitious paranoiac, I gradually became aware of a subtle pattern of fate. Anything I started seemed to be the ending of something. Schools I attended, places I visited, or various individuals I came across all seemed on the verge of collapse, but were followed by an abrupt shift to a startling new beginning even perhaps "a new world order." As far as personal patterns go (and patterns, you'll see, are lines of convergence and divergence as events play out over a span of time) mine was to begin at the tail of the old.

Is my immersion into qigong, thus a corollary? Is it my fate to usher in the poignant twilight re-emerging from the long corridor of ancient times? Is it the call of the ancients to their native son to serve as an emissary between the old, old wisdom and modern science? One thing is for certain: qigong saved my life and strengthen my body and soul to withstand the toxic side effects of chemotherapy. With my cancer cured, my body and mind regenerated, I am ready to begin transmission. This is the grateful message that I cast into the ether, a message from the masters whose consciousness accordingly still resides at the peak of Mount Taisan: Qi is the alchemy of healing.

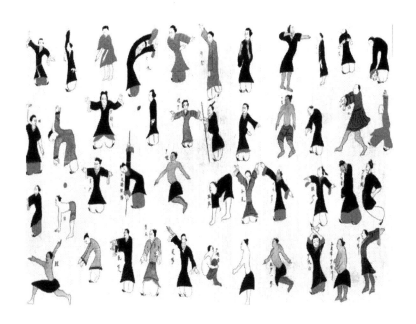

CHAPTER SIX: THE CANCER WARRIOR

Madame Gou Lin started simply to find a way of curing the ravage of her ovarian cancer. In the end, she discovered Medical Qigong and succeeded not only in eradicating her cancer but also helped millions of cancer patients in the world.

Consciousness is the only unifying reality and the greatest mystery of all.—Buddha.

WHAT EXACTLY IS A CANCER WARRIOR?

How the cosmos floats like a strand of wispy cloud across the vast expanse of consciousness. Within a single moment of recollection are infinite possibilities of expression.

To begin with, I can tell you that I was drafted into its file and rank by fate. A cancer warrior breaks out of the passivity of being a "survivor"—the state of mind that perceives cancer as a blight to endure. It requires one to engage in hand-to-hand combat, a fight literally to the death. The warrior gathers one's allies and stockpiles an arsenal of medicine in the guise of nutrition, exercise and meditation to battle the mad, dark twin within. The battlefield is our body and we are the General of our battalion.

To begin this war on cancer, we must first devise a strategy. Firstly, know thy enemy and oneself in order to assure victory. The question is not *what* is cancer but *who*. We must study it like a person's biography as each cancer has its own personality and inherent traits. Delving deep into the recesses of its long hazy past, we trace the ancient genealogy of its ancestors, the unfamiliar landscape of its origins, and strange nether catacombs where it hides. This dark encroaching shadow threatens to drain our life and overrun our biology by incessant hyperactive replication.

Your foremost ally in this campaign against cancer is your oncologist—your Lieutenant. Oncologists are a unique breed of physician as they are part scientist, part healer and part alchemist. It is they who concoct the potent chemo. Their strategy against these almost invisible microbial forces (cell migration, supra-cellular division) is to contain, destroy and constantly attenuate the battlefront. Cancer has a chimeric, shape shifting nature. It is not a sickness of infection or degeneration; but, at its core, cancer is the successful hyper-growth of abnormally mutated cells creating an evil parasitic doppelgänger inside one's own body. In order to combat this dark twin, your Lieutenant (the oncologist) must judge whether he is inflicting a lethal dose of chemotherapeutic agents upon the cancer cells *or* the patient. The oncologist will titrate the poison to the limit one's body can bear, in other words, to the point of death. Fundamentally, this strategy is based on the premise that healthy normal cells will regenerate and repair themselves better than the mutated cancerous cells.

Foremost in your arsenal is your mind with its totality of consciousness. Being a Buddhist, I have experienced the power of the mind in healing. After a difficult childbirth, my wife's cesarean section turned into a fourteen-hour surgery. After a transfusion that replaced three times the units of her blood and high doses of blood clotting fluids, the bleeding still would not stop. It was only when she heard the first cry of our newborn daughter that the bleeding instantaneously ceased. Later on, we named our daughter, Singha, for her singing healed her mother on the day she was born. Therefore, with a positive mental intention of the battle's outcome, you will invoke the heavens to assist you.

The tactical advantage that you possess is that cancer cells are weaklings; they are easily damaged and destroyed. Their only strength is their ability to replicate. Herein lies the strategy of chemotherapy and radiation: by administering a blanket destructive assault on the entire body, most of the cancer cells and as well as our normal cells will be damaged. As with most mutations, the copies are usually less robust than the normal ones. Cancer relapse occurs because the spray of chemotherapy or radiation missed a few hidden cancer cells as they were not in a highly active phase. Sometimes the treatment itself can cause more cellular mutations and thus create new cancer in the future. Therefore, it is critical that cancer treatment includes preventive measures both during and post-chemo/radiation treatment. As with any battle, prevention of the onslaught before it happens is superior to engaging in combat.

This is a manual on the art of combating cancer. In the Book of War by Sun-tze, three stages of the warrior's mindset are described:

1.   Utter ignorance of oneself and one's enemy.

2.   Knowing oneself but ignorant of the enemy.

3.   Knowing oneself as well as your enemy.

In most wars of early Western history, the first stage is more prevalent. One of the most glaring examples of such utter ignorance is illustrated in the infamous battle between Alexander and the Persian King Darius III. Alexander usurped power of Persia in a series of decisive battles, most notably the battles of Issus and Gaugamela by overthrowing King Darius III and subsequently conquering the entire Persian Empire. Darius fell into the first warrior's mindset due to the ignorance of his own military strength as well as his lack of reconnaissance regarding Alexander's new initiative—the cavalry in wing formation. The etiquette of nobility at the time required Darius to go to war with a full accompaniment of musicians and dancers to entertain him during battle. Darius viewed the Greek army as nothing more than a bunch of barbarians no better than annoying vermin deserving to be squashed. In addition, Darius had a habit of beheading messengers bearing bad news from the front. Therefore, by the time he personally took command, his head was filled with news of victory fabricated by intelligent messengers who wished to save their necks.

Like Darius, this is the unfortunate state people find themselves in who sternly believe in their idiosyncratic means to heal cancer. Without in-depth knowledge of their own cancer stage, type and chosen therapy's effectiveness, they have already lost the battle. And sometimes in a frontal assault, some of carcinomas (especially the cancerous stem cells) will come up from behind and attack from a hidden location.

Know yourself as well as your opponent. Your oncologists are your most battle hardened and experienced frontline. They have devoted their entire lives to studying and treating cancer and some have treated hundreds of cases. Hence, if possible, it is best to find an oncologist that specializes in your particular type of cancer. Learn as much as you can from him/her regarding the cause, treatment and post-treatment protocols. However, do not rely solely on your oncologist and become a passive participant in this epic battle. Remember, you are the emperor of this war. Know that oncologists are scientists who base their healing strategies on material science and clinical data. Their treatment protocols are based on research and positive results from previous clinical trials. However, specialists have built-in limitations, once you step out of their laser-trained field of expertise. Therefore, your oncologist cannot adequately advise you regarding diet, exercise or mindfulness. You have to assemble your own team to guide you in these areas. This book aims to point you in the right direction, sharing fundamental tools to use in your battle against cancer. I salute you from one warrior to another. May the heavens be with you.

OPPONENT: CANCER

Your opponent is not just the parasitic cancerous cells growing in your body but also the cancer inductive environment in which you are immersed. These are the pathogenic environmental factors (PEF).

Radioactive PEF: For example, Russian citizens who lived in or near Chernobyl were soaked in radiation and therefore have significant incidents of cancer.

Electronic PEF: We are surrounded by electromagnetic fields that induce stress on our cells. Stress serves as an immune suppressor and will inhibit an immune response toward cancer cells.

Chemical PEF: Recently New York City banned the use of trans-fats in all restaurants due to their toxic effect on the body. This saturated fat can result in a host of serious illnesses such as heart disease, asthma and cancer.

Emotional and mental PEF: Living in a psychologically stressful situation is akin to living on top of a toxic radioactive dump. Constantly living under a state of distress induces an inhibited immune system. Clinical data has shown that chronic depression will completely shut down the immune system. People who suffer from chronic depression have higher incidence of serious infection as well as cancer. On the other hand, there has never been a clinical study on cheerfulness acting as a shield against cancer. However, there is a famous case of the writer, Norman Cuisine who laughed himself to health by watching Marx Brothers comedies. He literally laughed his way out of an incurable sickness.

Biochemical PEF: The insulin factor has been shown to induce an inflammatory response in the body, resulting in allergies, infection and hypersensitivity. In this state of inflammation, the body's cells go into cell division hyper drive thus, increasing the chance of cancerous mutations.

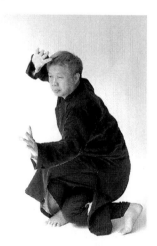

YOUR ARMY AND ARSENALS AGAINST CANCER

As already mentioned above, your oncologist is your frontline commander. He is like an alchemist in titrating the lethal chemotherapy dosage based on your response, as well prescribing rescue medicine to combat the side effects of the chemical mainlined into your veins. In my opinion, chemotherapy is more akin to alchemy than chemistry. Its process is still quite shrouded in mystery. Why it works for some patients and utterly fails for others is beginning to be uncovered by DNA mapping of various individual cancer cells. In a recent study, a single category of lymphoma yielded 80 distinctive genetic variants of cancer cells. It is the particular genetic makeup of cancer that predicts how the patient responds to standard chemotherapy treatment. New designer drugs are synthesized, developed in labs to specifically target cancer cells. Thus, if you have a type of cancer that responds especially well to chemotherapy, your chances of recovery are quite high.

Diet: Phytonutrients (or phytochemicals) are a most effective weapon against cancer. Phyto is Greek for plant; therefore, phytonutrients are chemical substances we absorb from plants. Unlike vitamins and minerals that are essential for cell growth and development, phytonutrients are not necessarily needed in the same way, but they may help prevent disease and make our bodies work more harmoniously. These chemicals have evolved on the Earth to us protect against cancer. Dr. G once informed me that it is not just by accident that substances such as curcumin, soy and garlic, amongst a host of others, are central elements in the cooking of diverse civilizations. Because of this discovery there is a whole new approach to the assimilation of these cancer-fighting phytochemicals: isolate particular nutrients when needed, and combine various nutrients to make a genuine attack on the chain of events that cause malignancies in one out of every three Americans. Under the masterful guidance of Dr. G, I consumed exclusively phytonutrient rich vegetables and supplements during my cancer treatment phase. Even after completing my cancer treatments, I have continued with these regimens and have expanded my diet to include other vegetables as well. Moreover, I still maintain a very strict sugarless diet to maintain a steady insulin level and to prevent a multitude of excessive sugar consumption diseases.

Here are some common vegetables rich in Phytonutrients: Green Tea, broccoli, cabbage, onion, celery, sesame seeds, olive oil, grape seed extracts. Eat a generous helping of them daily; as Dr. G reminds his patients frequently, "Phytonutients are great, but you need to eat a large quantity in order for them to be affective in fighting cancer. Thus, having one serving of broccoli a day is not enough to actively strengthen your immune system. Therefore, I recommend all my cancer patients to take concentrated supplements."

A word of caution: Please do not rush out to your local health-food store and buy those supplements without the guidance from a physician or a nutritionist.

Below is one of my favorite snacks of all time:

La Petite Phytonutrient snack:

3 stalks of organic celery stalks

1 Tsp of sesame oil for dipping sauce

Wash and cut the celery stalk into palm-size length. Dip it into a saucer of sesame oil and enjoy. (Caution: Raw vegetables should not be consumed during your chemo-cycle treatment period. Chemotherapy depletes your body of its immunity making you prone to infection.)

MIND/SPIRIT/CONSCIOUSNESS

Mind, body and spirit are integral to our treatment and one of the most powerful weapons in our fight against cancer. At the sublime level of deep meditation, Buddhist monks unify mind, body and spirit into the singular state of pure Being. In this state, it is possible that the mind's intention (included within the whole) can influence the outcome of ordinary events in physical reality. Buddhists call this consciousness only reality or the realm of form. For example, our body, the mountain, the molecules, sun, moon, planets and stars are but condensed states of consciousness. Hence, matter is consciousness; consciousness is matter.

At Princeton University, my alma mater, an ingenious experiment was conducted where college students were asked to mentally choose one of two images either a cowboy or an Indian. The experiment showed that the mind's intention (mental influence) directed the appearance of the desired image on the computer screen even though it was generated by a randomized event algorithm. The resulting data from these studies was statistically significant from instances of a non-intentionally directed outcome. Simply put, if the college student intended to have more cowboy images, then the outcome shifted toward more cowboys displaying on the computer monitor. It is similar to a red gum ball popping out of a machine filled with many possible other colored gum balls merely because a child wishes for the red one. I have often witnessed such events and parents of course logically explain to the child that the relationship between his/her intention and the resulting outcome is mere coincidence, thereby affirming the prevalent belief in the separation of mind and matter.

Sometimes in a deep meditative state, I can almost hear the anguished cries of multitudinous cancer patients calling forth a champion to lead them out of their suffering. My cancer now healed, I feel the urgency to share from the inside the way to activate this inherent spontaneous healing capacity. This is my destiny, my dharma and karma. Like Captain Ahab who caste forth a filament to catch the Great White whale, I feel this truth so vividly that I can nearly reach out and touch this potential cancer cure.

At times, as I practice the healing Qigong walk in the park, I have an uncanny sense of a long line of cancer patients following behind me. This experience illustrates the Taoist concept of *mind projection*. Taoists view time and events as one complete dynamic whole; the past, present and future are, in essence, existing in a extra dimension beyond time and space. Unlike the sequential progression of a film, this understanding of time would be a dynamic state of interactive shifts and changes. Therefore, in this example, the power of mind projection can impact the life of a single individual, me. However, I can choose either to accept my karma or not. By embracing my healing journey, I am compelled to learn about cancer. I feel the balance and rightness of the path. The ancient vow of the Buddha who sought liberation from the pain and suffering of life, death, sickness and old age, not only for himself, but also for the salvation of all sentient beings, resounds within me. I hope to follow in his footsteps.

MOVEMENT/EXERCISES/QIGONG

"I did not set out to discover the anticancer qigong; rather, it came out of my own desperation to find a cancer cure for myself."

—Gou Lin, a talk to a class of anticancer qigong teachers
at the Lavender Bamboo Grotto, Beijing. (1970)

When Gou Lin discovered that she had ovarian cancer, she was a plain, roly-poly woman in her late 50's. Her prescription sunglasses were the only exotic feature on her round moon face. She was a professor at the National Art Institute and in her student days, she studied with the old grandmaster of brush painting, Ci Bao Xia. As a young girl, she won the local province's first marathon and studied martial arts with her grandfather which included hard, strenuous qigong.

For Madame Guo, the pioneering cancer warrior, cancer was, above all, profoundly personal. It burnt within her. In the brown-obsidian iris of her newborn granddaughter's eyes, Gou Lin saw that an amorphous, malignant Mara was pursuing humanity from the shadowy depths of the Precambrian sea. Gou Lin surmised that cancer was born from the process of evolution. The final installment of humanity's epic battle is a saga of millennia and this foe was meant to be conquered.

She had survived World War II, the Japanese War and a civil war thus, with bone-chilling certainty, she had faith that nature would grant the antidote to this most insidious, deadly nemesis. The meticulous alchemist would use herself as her own guinea pig in her laboratory. "Look," she might whisper, "this shapeless lump of neoplasia exhibits an anaerobic mode of metabolism." In a Petri dish, a grape-size carcinoma taken from her own body showed a mode of metabolism lacking oxygen, elevated glucose consumption, carbon monoxide and high lactic acid production.

Gou Lin's central tenets:

First—Observe! The fighter who averts her eyes on the angry pulsating lava mass has lost the war.

Second—Experiment! Knowledge of the internal anatomy of cancer is the entryway to denuding the many heads of the hydra. Most cancer patients, panic-stricken, fumble in viscid ignorance as they grasp at the latest fad of cancer cure: grape seeds, scorpion stings, vegetarianism, Macrobiotic diets…

Third—Practice qigong! Harnessing the intrinsic energy/Qi within our bodies will serve as the army to decimate the cancerous cells and restrict its exponential growth.

Fourth—Endurance. With a dedicated daily regimen rising at the crack of dawn to begin her qigong walk, Gou Lin was able to eradicate and cure her cancer. After undergoing six surgeries to remove the cancerous tissue, she committed herself to this new lifestyle. "By the sixth time I entered the operating room, I told my body that this was the last time I would put it under the surgeon's scalpel. If I survived this surgery, I vowed to heal myself with the new qigong that I recently discovered. The surgery would buy me the time I needed to put my qigong into action." Gou Lin recalled to a group of cancer patients during her rounds at the Beijing People's hospital oncology ward. She kept this vow and her cancer never recurred. Now, over 100 million people practice her qigong.

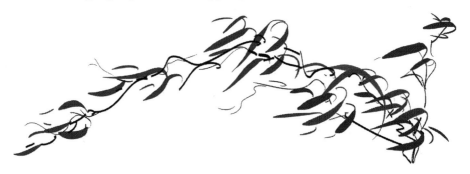

JOURNEY TO THE LAVENDER BAMBOO GROTTO

As a young intern in a Traditional Chinese Medical hospital, you are about to begin a stroll down Beijing's Lavender Bamboo grotto; you slip on the cotton bottom Kung Fu shoes, adjust the collar of your linen shirt, switch off the lights in the house and step out into the pre-dawn darkness. You wait for your guide, a cancer patient of yours, and together you crisscross the torturous tiny alleyways with their crumbling stone houses standing guard in silence. Having anticipated that you will need to record Gou Lin's words, you drop a small tape recorder in your pocket. You rub your eyes, yawn with your hands covering your mouth so as not to seem rude to your young patient—and find yourself spiraling down a cochlea of memories and snapshots:

Flash! A young mother weeps. She just discovered that she has stage IV metastatic breast cancer. You have been treating her almost since the beginning when she came to you for complementary treatment. She was cradling her newborn in her arms. She was worried that her milk would not be good for the baby. You assured her that it is still good; cancer is not transmittable. She smiled ruefully, "At least I am at still good for something."

Flash! The crush of chemo turned this vital young mother into a gaunt skeleton. Her baby is still clinging to her, but with the toxic treatment, she can no longer feed the child with her own breast milk. The young mothers of her village donated their extra milk for the baby. Now, she feeds her baby with other women's milk holding the bottle with the tenderness of a butterfly. "Mama will row you to the silver river by the moon," she sings an old lullaby. Your search far and wide for an acupuncture treatment for cancer has yielded dismal results. All you can do is reduce her pain.

Flash! Miraculous, she bounced back in one day and shouted aloud, "My cancer is in remission!?" Her oncologist said that this was so, and he was, frankly, quite surprised as well. Words tumbled out in a jumble about how she had cried alone on a park bench while an elderly woman passed by with fluid grace, and she was compelled to follow the old woman who told her how she had cured her own cancer with this walk… you check her pulse at the wrist and feel the strength of her blood; you looked into her eyes and find a fighter standing defiant against the foe: cancer. You laugh and cry with her and share in her exuberance. So, you decide to find out all about the old woman, this cancer warrior, for yourself.

After dodging a hair-raising torrent of maniacal bicyclists racing down the Boulevard, you enter an oasis of bamboo swaying in the morning breeze. Dazed, you follow her through the gate toward a pavilion in the middle of the park. About two yards to your right, you spot a group of people already gathered around a chubby young man.

"Ha, ha, you know the only thing cancer is afraid of is laughter. You can literally laugh away your cancer." The group leader cackles. So true. Laughing is better than crying, because when you laugh, you are sucking in gallons of air.

You wonder how could this be a group of cancer patients, the survivors of a most fatal disease. How could they laugh? You find yourself drifting toward the group. Don't settle with just surviving cancer, you want to defeat it, beat it so that it will never come back.

"Be a warrior," a rotund woman, gently waddles forward to speak to the group. She wears the typical homespun short-sleeved blouse with a pattern of little plum blossoms. Her soft, melodious voice hypnotically draws you inexplicably toward her. You suddenly realize that she is the founder and creator of anticancer qigong. In her presence, an electric current seems to run through the circle of cancer patients gathering around her. As you draw near, you feel the awe that you had when you flew for the first time above the hinterlands of the Siberian tundra. Startled by your own reaction, you take a step back and wonder.

"My fellow warriors," she calls out, disturbing a flock of iridescent throated doves cooing on the lawn so that they flutter and scatter, airy puffs while tiny umbrellas of dandelion swirl in the autumn breeze. "We have us a battle to win, don't we, now."

"Don't we now, don't we," the crowd softly chanted and echoed.

You have read in medical journals that most cancers are incurable; a cancer patient could only bear and survive both the treatment and the disease, hence the name: cancer survivor. Since the dawn of time, shamans, pundits, alchemists, doctors, scientist, emperors, dictators, priests, puritans and Philistines have proclaimed that cancer is a suppuration of blood, a fossilized mass like a crustacean's carapace and could not be cured. It could only be endured while one waited for the other shoe to drop: recurrence. So, you are somewhat hesitant, but you tell yourself that, the grand architect of Chinese medicine, the Yellow Emperor wrote, "Most pathologies have their primary cause in our being out of balance with the earth, the sun and the moon..." and with a shiver of trepidation you step out to interview the great master, the cancer warrior, Gou Lin.

Soon, you find you are having trouble catching up with the group, as they take off in their languorous qigong walk; as swift as a summer breeze, they pass a shimmering pond with a shoal of jeweled emerald goldfish immobile in their wide-eyed dream. *How could this be, left in the dust by a group of cancer patients?* A few stretches later, you fall upon a narrow passage among elephantine trunks of jade-green bamboo. And as you trudge uphill, panting and flush, you spot a lone figure briskly circling the pond almost in a run.

"Ah, that's Xiao Chan, who had been rejected by most hospitals as a hopeless case; his tumor had grown to the size of a small melon." Gou Lin points out. "I had to show him a fast walking qigong to restrict the cancerous growth in his body."

Years later, you track the life of Xiao Chan; his cancer has been completely eradicated, and he returns to his beloved native land, Outer Mongolia, where he started a branch of anticancer qigong and thus, quickly became a minor local celebrity.

An eternity later, it seems, you chance upon the bright idea of taping an interview with Gou Lin about her discovery of her unique qigong. After sidling up to the pioneer of anticancer qigong, you ask her a few questions:

Madame, how would you describe the process which lead to your discovery of anticancer qigong? Without skipping a beat, she replies, "Cancer has an emotional and psychological aspect to it. At the time I discovered I had uterine cancer, it was the start of the Cultural Revolution; my husband was purged from the university and exiled to the farmland for labor reform camp. During that period, I was teaching at the art department. Being a professor in China, I was given preferential medical care, and at the time the best, viable therapy protocol was a radical hysterectomy." As you listen, though you know you really mustn't, you can't help but mentally recall the history of clinical cancer treatments.

William Stewart Halsted, the surgeon whose name was forever linked with the concept and practice of radical surgery, accidentally stumbled into the world of physical medicine. He rebelled against his father by avoiding the family garment business and became a surgeon. To refine his surgical craft, Halsted traveled to Europe to study the latest techniques. After apprenticing with several world-renowned surgeons, the young Halsted gained the tremendous skills in dissecting and excising tumors from cancer patients.

In search of a framework for cancer treatment, Halsted had a sudden insight that cancer was like an infectious growth—a hideous parasitic overactive fungi (or *a little flower of horror*) that threatened to eat the body from within. He took a radical approach by cutting away as much of the infected tissue as possible to prevent its insidious spread. However, surgeons at that time lacked potent anesthesia for their operations. Halsted had to wait until 1884, when cocaine was discovered as a form of fast acting anesthesia. In a few years, armed with the anesthetic and meticulous surgical skills, he achieved a meteoric rise as a surgeon who could rescue patients from the brink of death. Nevertheless, no matter how carefully Halsted tried to remove all traces of the cancerous tissue, many of his patients eventually relapsed after the initial operation. Frantic and desperate to save his patients, Halsted extended the fungi analogy to the notion that cancer spread from a radiating center. He would cut away whole infected breast cavities, eradicating the underlying healthy tissue beneath the breast, amputate major muscle groups of the shoulder and in some cases even the collar bone and ribs. Essentially, he butchered the complete breast, henceforth the term "radical mastectomy." Paradoxically, his patients faithfully wrote notes of profound gratitude for his "life saving" procedures. Unfortunately, (or fortunately), later clinical data proved that such extreme, excessive surgical techniques did not extend the patient's life span.

Suddenly a flash from early Bible studies comes to mind: "And if thine eye offends thee, pluck it out…"

In a domino effect stretching over the span of a century, the scalpel of Halsted's Chinese disciple cut into Gou Lin as her radical hysterectomy no doubt followed Halsted's protocol. After six unsuccessful surgeries with the last one so drastic that she was in a coma for days, Gou Lin was discharged and told by her doctors "to settle her affairs". But she was not ready to die just yet…

Jostled from your reverie, a young man approaches, his spiral walk centers upon you, and he touches your shoulder with a gentleness almost verging on tenderness.

"Madame Gou saved my life. Most of the hospitals in Beijing refused to accept my hopeless case as the cancer was in its 4th stage…there is no 5th stage in cancer." His laugh almost seemed like a cough as he ruminated how near he had skirted death's edge.

"But she told me that she had great faith in her qigong's effectiveness in arresting the metastasis of carcinomas. I must completely dedicate every moment to diligent practice." Ah, how true it is! You saw the shimmering light dancing in his brown irises like sunflowers bending toward the sun. All this time, Gou stood by and shuffled the floor embarrassed by all the praise from her loyal students. After all, she did save their lives. By then a small congregation had gathered to hear his tale and each started to relate their own testimonies, their individual harrowing encounters with cancer. One leathery, wizened man shared that he had already written his last will before he left his village. He sought out Gou Lin in a last-ditch effort to save his life from late stage metastasized lung cancer. His children accompanied him to Beijing to fulfill his bucket list. After three months of practicing Gou Lin's qigong, his cancer was in remission; his children were ecstatic and decided to relocate their families to the capital. One of his daughters even graduated from Gou Lin's qigong teacher's training course. She now led several groups of cancer patients in various oncology wards.

You are so stunned by positive reports that you ask Gou Lin whether there are any clinical scientific investigations validating her qigong's capability to heal and cure cancer.

"Yes, a scientist from the Beida oncology unit came out to gather clinical data from my cancer patients who practice qigong vs. a control group in hospitals. He collected over 600 cases over a period of three years, and his results showed an 85% improvement in life extension of the cancer patients who practiced the qigong; and 25% among the qigong population were completely cured. The results were so significant that he persuaded the Health Ministry to start a national program to make the qigong available in all oncology wards in China.

"I personally trained over 1,000 qigong teachers and now they will scatter to the four corners of the world to go forth and spread beauty and light…" You suddenly realized that Gou is quoting from Shakespeare's Sonnets: *Go forth and spread beauty and light.*

To understand the principles of how qigong can serve as a Complementary Therapeutic practice alongside the traditional medical treatments of chemotherapy, radiation and surgery, we must visit the three thousand-year-old tradition of Chinese medicine. In the following chapters, we will explore some fundamentals of Chinese medicine.

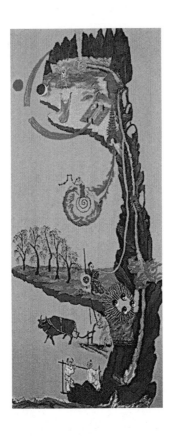

CHAPTER SEVEN:
TRADITIONAL CHINESE MEDICINE

"In antiquity, the people were simple and so were their diseases, hence it would suffice to perform incantations and magical dances to vanquish the evils from their bodies." Yellow Emperor Treatise in Medicine (2598 BC)

Traditional Chinese Medicine (TCM) originates from a civilization and culture that appeared thousands of years before the Egyptians built their pyramids, or the Sumerians collected their clay tablets in libraries. To this day, TCM and its practice continues to be a vibrant part of an enormous network of healing culture. It is the beating heart of healthcare for 1.6 billion Chinese and promotes a balanced lifestyle to assure wellbeing, health and healing. The essence of Chinese medicine derives from the same source as all other disciplines whether it be philosophy, government, ethics, or science... The Tao is that source, the spontaneous nature of the cosmos—nothing more, nothing less.

Simply put, health is living in accord with the Tao, the natural order and flow of the universe. This principle, in my opinion, radiates continually with crystalline clarity. Human lives are dependent on the terrain they inhabit, the weather that surrounds them, the cycles of life and finally the collective environment. We are influenced by the subtle effects of lunar phases and the explosive astronomical events of sun spots. At other times, nature throws humans devastating blows such as the case of hurricanes or tsunamis. Again, revisiting the Chinese medical classic, *The Yellow Emperor's Treatise on Internal Medicine,* (3000 B.C.) the descriptions attributed to the ancient sagely monarch of diseases and treatments still resound with such poignancy.

"...In antiquity, the people were simple and so were their diseases, hence it would suffice to perform incantations and magical dance to vanquish the evils from their bodies."

—Yellow Emperor's Treatise on Internal Medicine

However, in our modern times, there is no such luck! Pathogens, I sense, are evolving in parallel with the progress of human civilization. No longer will it suffice to chant and dance to chase the pernicious humors away. Modern diseases require a vast array of technology and modeling to give healers a guiding theory and principles to combat the ravages of diseases such as cancer. Inch by inch, or so it seems, ancient Chinese doctors peeled away the exterior symptoms of cancer as they surfaced in the form of tumors, pain and fever. As a result, the innards of the body were revealed: bones, organs and intestines.

Cancer is the evil twin of fecundity and dark sorcerer conjuring shape shifting maladies. These are the ninja assassins lurking in the very fabric of our genetic structure or DNA. And yet, sidling along this shadowy killer is potential victory.

Pathology is a battle between the forces of good and evil. When the evils of environmental forces such as, heat, cold, wind, aridity, humidity and fire infiltrate us, they join forces with our preexisting internal malaises which include depression, rage, stupor, anxiety and obsession. Together, they overwhelm our immune Qi (the good force) and thus, the spark of cancer begins. The cancerous seeds occupy regions where one's energy is stagnant and congested like log-jammed pools overgrown with algae and Spanish moss.

"When there is stagnation of Qi/energy and blood, it creates an internal landscape ripe for the infiltration of external pernicious factors. Within these pools of stagnation pathogens take root and grow. Thus cancer has two aspects, the carcinomas in situ and the systemic stagnant network that enables cancer's propagation. (Cancer research has shown that in order for cancer cells to migrate, i.e. the metastasized cells mutate taking on the ability to stimulate blood vessel growth and therefore, supply cancer's manic growth.) Hence, cancer requires a two-pronged attack: destroy and eradicate the tumors in conjunction with a restoration of the free flow of Qi at the stagnated network."

—from a talk from teachers' training by Gou Lin at the Medical Qigong seminars. (1984)

River metaphors are imprinted on the Chinese psyche for the Yellow River, no doubt, influenced the nascent evolution of the people and its civilization. Therefore, the fundamental principle of pathology is our life-stream in distress: stagnant water choked with poisonous growth, a flood overwhelming our defenses, or acrid draught burning through our flesh. Hence, the attributes of sickness are fiendish malevolence described as dampness, feverish fire, acrid draught, bone-chilling cold, turbulent winds. Cancer, being the most powerful magus, possesses all these malignancies. Hence, in combating cancer, the patient is catapulted into the role of river-tamer, dredging out the pitch-dark muck from the energy pathways, unblocking stagnation with acupuncture and qigong, fighting against the eroding nutrients with herbs. As you can see, the rescue remedies fit within the watery metaphors neat as a silken glove.

ANATOMY OF OUR ENERGY BODY

Quite auspiciously, there exists an anatomy text in the guise of a landscape painting that can guide us towards a rudimentary knowledge of TCM. The image is a symbolic diagram incorporating humans, the cosmos, sun, moon, stars, trees, mountain, ocean, and subterranean streams. The land-scape draws on the usual imagery of Chinese landscape paintings: mountains, glacial peaks, tumbling waterfalls, underground streams and at the very bottom, the ocean. However, the landscape emerges as a microcosm of human existence as it warps and weaves the sublime interaction of agents and forces that govern human life. The painting ingests the human body, processes it and spits it out. Our physical anatomy is transformed into a floating mountain emerging out of a cobalt-blue ocean, encircled by the eternal twin luminaries of sun and moon.

Originally, this painting was procured from a rock carving on a cliff face. Inscribed on the carving is a text that proclaims that the origin of the rock hewn image was based on a scroll discovered accidentally by a court physician during one of his annual summer sojourns. On a visit to a Taoist monastery, he accidentally came upon a dusty scroll hidden in a crevice in the cloister's library. He immediately realized that he had found a rare long lost map of the human body. The physician was more than a simple court official; he was also an adept in inner alchemy, the esoteric art of immortality. Perhaps he was torn by a selfish desire to preserve the knowledge for himself and his family versus a selfless intent of generosity toward humankind. Nevertheless, he kept the scroll secret and only near the end of his life did he reveal it to the world by chiseling the image on the mountain peak.

The inscription read: "...since the discovery of the scroll, I have greatly benefited from the knowledge of the inner anatomy and hence, I share this secret with future generations..." Such a magnanimous deed allowed the scroll to become the de facto Taoist's alchemical 'bible'.

During one of my sojourns in China, I climbed up a thousand steps to reach the top of White Cloud Mountain. Exhausted, I literally stumbled upon this very map etched into the mountain side. I instantly recognized it as an energetic map of the human body.

As we enter the map of this enchanted landscape, we are guided by ensorcelled beings: a sage, a monk, and finally an archetypal child. At the center of this image is the most intriguing crystalline cave where the child dances the sacred steps of the Big Dipper entombed in a womb-like lambent light. This cave is a symbol for the heart, the seat of consciousness. Contrasted with illustrations of western anatomical texts depicting blood red arteries, striated muscle bundles or ghostly white skulls forever grinning emaciated smiles; personally, I prefer the Chinese one.

In studying this image, we are reminded that humans are small creatures, but intrinsically related to the Earth and the whole fabric of life. We, in our homocentric daily preoccupations (running to catch a train or driving the children to soccer games and ballet classes) are beset by a thousand cuts. We have lost sight of the impending dark storm brewing on the horizon and Chinese medicine is prodding us to look more closely at the approaching cumulus clouds. To live in harmony with nature, we have to explore the hidden forces and principles that govern life.

To begin this journey of self-discovery, we must first acquire a key to this internal landscape: our own microcosm. This key is the fundamental unifying principle of the substance called Qi. All living things and organic substances are but Qi in its manifold materialization and appearance. Paradoxically, Qi remains elusive like the Cheshire cat only appearing when it smiles; thus, we can witness the functioning of Qi only in action, but never the 'Cheshire cat' itself. Hence, the whole cosmos is one huge, gigantic kaleidoscope of Qi appearances as it takes on infinite roles but is never itself. So, in studying the inner map of our body, the mountain is qi, the ocean is qi, the monk is qi: it is all Qi. And this is the key to understanding the inner map.

A TOUR OF TRADITIONAL CHINESE MEDICINE

By fate or serendipity I was initially drawn towards studying neuroscience in college and became familiar with the anatomical structures of bones, muscles, and the metabolic processes of various organic systems such as endocrine or cardiovascular. But it was only when I encountered a fifteen hundred year old stone carving of a landscape with the shape of a human torso that I began to discover the hidden meaning of these structures and how they might reveal another dimension of our world. But in order to begin this journey, we must decide which aspects of Chinese Medicine we deem necessary.

This metaphoric landscape reveals the body's energetic functions. The two luminaries of the sun and moon are symbols for our eyes that allow light into the consciousness. The nine snowcapped peaks represent the nine major cortical brain functions. A glacial lake rests at the foothills of this Himalayan highland and from it a subterranean spring flows all the way down to the sea at the bottom symbolizing the cerebral spinal fluid as well as the spinal cord.

From this image I have learned the wiles of an innovative esoteric language of body and consciousness. A language whose twists and turns seems all too alien to our modern-day scientific orientation. One senses a luminous aura stripping away all the outer layers of physicality to reveal a single instant of an ephemeral existence; one begins to penetrate the elemental mystery of Being. A concealed infrastructure is made visible all at once through an image chiseled into stone; it is imprinted in my brain, superimposing itself everywhere and on everything.

To grasp this quintessential notion is our chance to become what my Chinese professor called a "wine soaked plum," in other words, a healer who sees the sublime, subatomic energy at the heart of medicine. Within this landscape, we walk hand-in-hand with the ancient shamans where life, sickness and death have become metaphors. We are shown how one lives and how one dies, opening up whole new vistas for the possibility of healing and even the ultimate remedy against the onslaught of our deadliest assassin, cancer.

For Chinese doctors, diseases are the dark side of life, the shadowy part of the moon, hiding and waiting to be revealed. We are born into a world of duality, comprised of the sunlight of health and the darkness of illness. Although we all wish to remain in the sunshine of wellness, if we live long enough, each of us will fall inevitably into the shadow of sickness and decline. The unavoidable karmic cycle of life, sickness, aging and death chains us in underlying fear and panic in face of unknown perils. From the TCM perspective, cancer is not only a mortal physical illness, but a metaphor and this is the most truthful way of regarding this disease—and the healthiest way of living it. The illness is a result of a multitude of contributing factors, which are often subtle and mostly unseen.

Yet it is hardly possible to take up one's residence in the realm of cancer unprejudiced by the lurid "facts" of blood tests, white blood cell counts, viral infection indexes and the ubiquitous scans. Each test slowly erodes the mystery of our humanity and the power of spontaneous healing. It is toward an elucidation of metaphors, and liberation from literal-minded thinking, that we begin this inquiry into the dark side of sickness and the body as a metaphor for a microcosm.

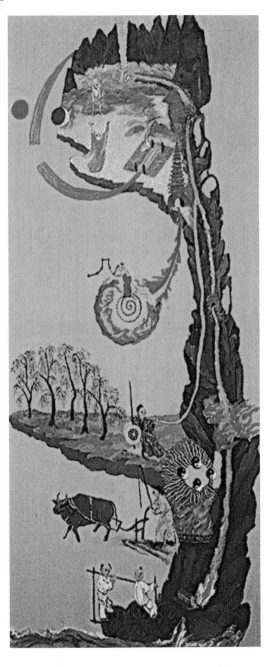

ENTERING THE INNER WORLD OF OUR BODY

The accompanying illustration is my rendition of the ink rubbing from the original stone relief. Hopefully, with the addition of color, the human organs' symbolic meaning will emerge and an intuitive grasp of the correlation between the natural elements and our own bodies is more easily realized.

To begin our foray into this mystical landscape, we must begin by locating our internal organs and biological systems depicted as external terrain. Mountain, river, sun, moon, oceans and the mythic demigods (the Sage, Monk, Jade Maiden, the Ox herder and the Immortal Red Lotus Child) transport us into unknown dimensions. We are on a fantastic voyage into the mythical realm of fairy tales and shamanic stories. Lets us, then, you and I, start at the peak of this sacred mountain and gradually descend downward.

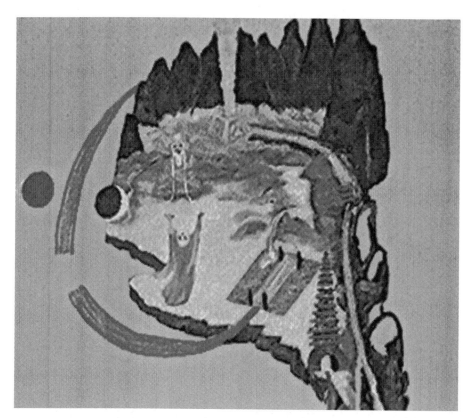

Imagine after an arduous climb, you finally arrive at the summit of Mount Everest at the very instant of sunset *and* moonrise. These twin luminaries appear simultaneously against the backdrop of a pale lapis lazuli sky. Without a doubt, this would be one of the most profound vistas ever seen in your life. The sun and moon balanced at the edge of the world, between heaven and earth. The masterful alchemist who created this iconic scene chose the sun and moon to represent the functions of our eyes. He deftly conceived the potential of our vision's pervasive influence on every aspect of our biological functions and cellular metabolism. Without sunlight, Earth would be plunged into darkness, and all life would be winked out of existence. Therefore, the allegory of sun and moon alludes to the essential stimulation allowing growth within our millions of cells and the healing power of light that penetrates our retinas. As the photons hit the rods and cones of the retinas, a tiny electrical pulse is generated, which travels along the optic nerves into the visual cortex at the back of the head. Incidentally, if we happen to take a nasty fall and bang our head, we often see a bolt of blinding white light as our visual cortex is stimulated directly from this blow.

Perhaps, informed by this biological process, the alchemist in meditation visualizes light penetrating the 'third eye' (the space between the eyes) and directs it backward into the head. Then he experiences the light pouring into and infiltrating every pore, organ and cell of the body. Hence, alchemical cultivation is replete with practices that mirror phenomena found in nature and our biology. The alchemical simulation of natural processes aims to achieve mastery of one's biology. One is then no longer subject to mere reflexes or unconscious reactions, but one becomes a participant through awareness and in the final stage, one may be able to intentionally direct the flow of energy and endocrine secretions. For instance, in the common sexual tantric practice of redirecting ejaculation, during orgasm, the male novice pulls up the perineum in order to prevent the seminal fluid from flowing outward and draws the precious creative liquid up to the spine and into the brain. This is one of the clearest illustrations of Taoist alchemy's mastery of biology and its attempt to reverse the downward flow. (A word of caution: this particular method is fundamentally flawed. The verbal teaching may have been truncated and hence, corrupted as it was passed down over many generations. Readers beware.)

Returning to the topic at hand, the very first alchemists were scientists and shamans interested in using minerals as catalysts to transmute the body, therefore transforming mutable mortals into changeless gold-like immortals. Since gold is considered an immutable substance (thus immortal) the forefathers of modern chemists experimented with mercury along with a few other minerals to make gold into a digestible form, an elixir called Jin Dan, 金丹, Golden Seed. By ingesting gold, these early alchemists hoped to absorb its immutable quality.

A branch of these mineral alchemists later spread through the trade route on the Silk Road and established an Arabic sect which subsequently influenced the medieval European courts and their nascent universities. The mythic Merlin is the West's most famous alchemist who mastered the ultimate redirection of the aging process and grew younger with each passing day. Thus, the Neolithic script of proto-Chinese for the sun, the prime force for life on Earth, is a circle drawn with a dot at the center and also stands for gold. In western astrology, the circle with a dot is a glyph for Sol and moreover represents the sun. The disciplines of Taoist alchemy and astrology are descendants of a common ancestor who had the audacity to stand against the wheel of death and challenge fate in an attempt to become God-like. As we can see, the Inner Landscape is not only a map of our body but also serves as a guidebook to lead us towards the process of transmutation, which unfortunately is still shrouded in symbolic codes and encryptions. Hence, only a living master with a key to decode and unlock this map will be capable to guide the neophyte along such a journey. However, due to centuries of turmoil, the collapse of dynasties and the recent Cultural Revolution in China, most, if not all the old masters have been either executed or have died without passing on their wisdom and teachings. It is then with some trepidation and sense of obligation to revive this ancient flow that I will attempt to unveil some of the secret teachings behind the Inner Landscape.

Fortunately, truth and wisdom cannot be hidden forever. The eminent psychologist, Francine Shapiro, discovered a form of cognitive and behavioral psychotherapy that uses the movement of the eyes to resolve post-traumatic stress syndromes called Eye Movement Desensitization and Reprocessing (EMDR). In 1987, she observed, during a walk in the park, that moving her eyes seemed to reduce the stress of disturbing memories. Considering her initial observations, she developed standardized procedures to maximize these effects, conducted further research and subsequently published a randomized controlled study in 1989 describing these beneficial results. EMDR is recommended as a front line therapy for trauma in numerous international psychological practice guidelines.

Intrigued by this modern discovery of eye movement's therapeutic effects, I came to realize that humans are a very visual species. We have culturally evolved to increasingly rely on visual imagery for communication as well as other aspects of our existence. This is very different from the animal kingdom living nocturnally or in forests, where the primary senses used for survival for both prey and predators are smell and hearing. For example, deer have terrible eyesight, they rely more on hearing and smell than vision. When a deer finally spots a lurking cheetah, it is already too late to escape. Therefore, Darwinian natural selection is a factor in the development of this attribute.

Subsequently, for inner alchemical practitioners, the eyes and seeing are imperative for movement. Seeing and sensing the direction of one's movement is essential for directing the flow of energy along the body in motion. In the practice of qigong, a form of 'Taoist yoga', series of physical postures, movements and visualizations becomes potent techniques for the elimination of stress and the secret of bringing light and life into our consciousness.

THE IMMORTAL CHILD

Envision the mythical Merlin, the most well-known alchemist of the West, with hooded eyes and pointed cap—the outline of his form recedes into the shadows. Perched on a rickety stool, a raven, dark-as-night, gawks guttural complaints and hops onto the long table while a single candle flickers, illuminating the cold stone tower. An insomniac, Merlin would often awaken at the witching hour of 3 AM, the hour of complete darkness with the moon vanished and morning sun not yet risen. Strangely, the magus with his possession of such vast stores of knowledge and wisdom accumulated throughout the many millennia was unable to comprehend the most basic human fear, mortality. In having achieved a life without end, this divine gift robbed him of the exaltation of living, the excitement of the fleeting moment. For a man whose life stretched on for eternity, existence had become an utter bore, and he felt alienated from humanity. Quite perversely, immortality had made his existence an endless repetitive drudgery. It was like a poor man suddenly given the Midas touch—the ability to turn everything into gold—completely losing any interest in wealth. Money would no longer hold any conceivable meaning. An everlasting life in an Earthly existence is a meaningless one; he laughed at this cosmic joke.

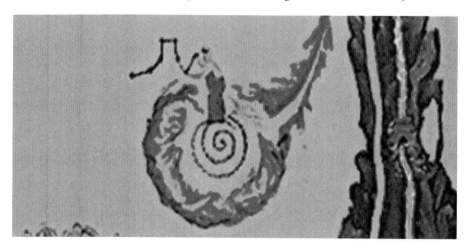

In the light of this insight, all parts of Merlin's life including the landscape, the movements of stars and revolving planets converge into a divine comedy of immortality played out in the mortal realm. His story serves as a maze, a puzzle where faint points of light delineate an unknown secret of inconceivable dimensions. His legendary life was riddled with reversals: his ability to grow younger as time passed and the eventual betrayal by his female acolyte, Morgan La Fay. Initially, she pretended to be a boy and then later seduced Merlin, who was by then all too willing to trade his godlike state for passion. La Fay eventually manipulated the magus by persuading him to teach her a spell that he could not unbind. This act of surrender and vulnerability was an ultimate demonstration of his love for her. Disenchanted with immortal life, Merlin was more than willing to relinquish his power to his one true love, even with full knowledge of her inevitable forthcoming betrayal. With this spell, Morgan La Fay trapped Merlin within the crystal cave and his regenerative life force was forever entombed.

Accordingly, the quest for immortality is where the life resides, not in its actual achievement. It is like a great painting wrapped in wax paper; the object possesses only a latent sublime beauty and therefore is only a most glorious masterpiece within the imagination. Such as it is with an immortal life, it only exists in potentiality and perhaps at another dimension of living. If ever one achieved such an incredible feat against insurmountable odds, the fruit of an everlasting life for the ordinary person would be most likely boredom.

Perhaps this is the metaphor of the Inner Landscape's young child dancing within the crystal cave at the heart. She still possesses an innocence of a perfect un-manifest potentiality, guided by the natural circling of the Big Dipper, pointing her towards the true North—the Self. Therefore, the alchemist's entrapment is the achievement of an objective immortality, a state of inert stability which in the end resembles a living death. Although everlasting life is an almost impossible feat, immortals at present only exist in myths and legends and therefore few seekers will ever have the opportunity to be disillusioned. One could say that the pursuit of immortality is more enlivening than attaining it, a perplexing dilemma indeed.

As legend has it, after the Yellow Emperor achieved immortality, he was obliged to leave the mortal world and so mounted his dragon at Mount Taishan and ascended to the heavens. His ministers desperately clung to the dragon's tail, but being Earth bound; they all inevitably fell back into the mortal realm. The men who fell to Earth were the ancient authors of many immortal texts and treatises. They wrote of their sorry attempts to grasp the tail of immortality.

This archetypal tale of the fall from grace or the expulsion from the Garden of Eden, points us toward a possible redemption, as this image in the inner landscape pairs the child in the heart with the Big Dipper—the symbol of the eternal. She dances in an ever inward spiral and traces the elliptical orbit of this constellation—a suggestion of a reversal leading into unknown dimensions.

Inspired by this archetypical image, the Seven Star Immortal child meditation is a fundamental mental cultivation for novices. In my experience, it is one of the most useful meditative processes to resolve childhood traumas. Hence, proceed with caution, and in the words of one infamous space captain, "Steady as she goes."

IMMORTAL CHILD MEDITATION

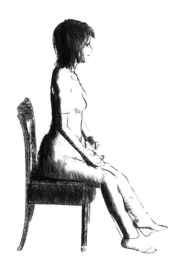

Overall, the meditation in this book can be done in any relaxed posture, whether reclined, seated or standing. This meditation is quite beneficial to do just before bedtime. After meditation, your body and mind will be in a state of great peace and comfort. You will awaken refreshed as if from a deep sleep. Before we embark on the meditation, it is crucial that we take a slight detour to prepare ourselves for the meditation. The following is a concise general guideline for meditation preparation.

GENERAL PREPARATION FOR TAOIST HEALING MEDITATION

I have frequently explained to my students that the practice of meditation is similar to playing the piano. Before any music can be played, the piano must be in tune; otherwise, even the greatest pianist performing a Bach masterpiece will sound like mud. Hence, it is essential that we begin any meditation with tuning the body.

In order to tune the body, we can start by just shivering, trembling and shaking out all the little fears inside, immerse yourself in this enhanced wonderful body awareness, and reveal your inner shadow, embracing it. Allow each droplet of despair or negative energy to be completely exorcised from your body and energy channels.

Next find a low stool or chair so that your feet can firmly rest on the floor. If you sit for long periods of time with your feet dangling in the air, it will cause the blood to drain down to the feet. Then spread your feet to the width of your shoulders—the common habit of crossing the legs while seated is appalling for your circulation, so avoid it like the kiss of death. Rest your hands on your knees with palms either down or up whichever you find more amenable. Now adjust your pelvis so that you are seated on the edge of the chair. (For the gentlemen, make sure your testicles are hanging freely and are not pressed against the chair—this is critical in freeing the sexual energy as well as avoiding the potential complication of impotence.) Seated in this way, you avoid resting your back against the chair; doing so will collapse the lumbar spine and compress the internal organs. Perhaps this way of sitting inspired the ancient masters to call it "sitting precariously." In ancient times, Taoist adepts would sit in this precarious fashion on the ledge of cliff overhangs, no doubt gazing into the yawning abyss below. After situating your body on the chair, locate a rising and falling motion in your lower abdomen, observe how the lower back, the lumbar vertebrae become free and undulate with each breath. This precarious sitting can also be practiced seated on a cushion. Take a small breath, and as you exhale, let your spine release like a strand of pearls hanging down.

After that, gently rotate your torso in a clockwise motion, starting with twenty-four rotations and then reverse the direction. Such a mild gyration will help to free and warm up the lumbar vertebrae. On the exhalation, drop the ribs as if you were folding in a beach umbrella, letting the ribs gather in. In order to facilitate this relaxation, place your palms on your ribs and softly stroke them to relax the intercostal muscles between the ribs. Furthermore, gently run your right palm over your stomach area to warm up the spleen and help its energy to flow. Soften your heart and chest. The chest should not be puffed up, nor should it be collapsed. Tap your fingers gently against your sternum. Sometimes excessive tension in the chest will cause the heart rate to quicken. In Medical Qigong therapeutic theory, softening the heart may slow down the heart rate. Now, continuing with the tuning of the body, imagine your head is like a buoy floating on water; this relaxes the cervical spine. At this moment, with a short inhalation, slightly tuck your chin as if nodding and saying yes to life. Touch the tip of your tongue to the roof of your mouth, the upper palate. (Variations: If you have a heart problem, touch the tongue to the bottom palate. If you would like to lose weight, let the tongue hang freely in the middle of the mouth without touching the palate.) Lower your eyelids, but keep them open to a tiny crack, so that you can see at a forty-five-degree angle down in front of you. The Taoist masters called this area "where the cow lies down." Do not close your eyes completely, for this may cause you to feel drowsy or your mind starts to wander. At last with your body tuned, your mind at ease, you are all set and ready to begin the Immortal Child Meditation.

IMMORTAL CHILD MEDITATION

The following is written as an audio guide for the meditation. As you read the sentences, just imagine my voice guiding you along the different stages of the meditation:

For the moment, with your eyes closed, take a few deep breaths. Breathe naturally without effort. It is as if after an epic climb to the top of Mount Blanc, you look out at the majestic panorama of snowcapped peaks, you sigh in deep relief, and breathe in the pure glacial air.

Now, allow your body to sink deep into the bed, and feel the solid surface supporting you. At this time, visualize a small child (perhaps four or five years old) seated in a lotus flower at the area of your heart near the Solar Plexus. At present, breath with this child. With each breath the child grows in size, but not in age. Keep breathing gently, until the child grows to the size of your whole body. When this occurs, let your senses reach out to this inner child and with imaginary arms embrace the child, and from your heart speak silently that everything is OK and that he/she has survived and will grow up to be successful and healthy. Maintain this state as long as you want, and sometimes you can even fall asleep embracing your own innermost self.

At this time, when you are ready to part with your inner child, softly say good-bye to the child and promise that you will come back. Now, imagine the child gradually shrinks in size until he/she becomes small enough for the lotus and enfold the child back into your heart. Then let your consciousness slowly rise up from the depths of your being into the present. Next rub your palms together to generate heat and place them over your chest, and feel the warmth spreading all over your body. Open your eyes to the outside world. Often, my students report that the world seems a bit brighter after the meditation. This meditation can be done daily or once in a while; it is entirely up to you. Never impose a discipline from the outside; it will merely lead to resistance and failure. Do the process because it feels good, and if you derive joy from it. In other words, there is no absolute right way of practicing.

In summary, the experience of this meditative practice could range from elation to great emotional release. When such experiences happen whether other images, sounds or other objects of the mind, you should not pay them heed, but instead treat them as part of the rolling landscape of a riverbank as you flow down the river. Don't attach or fixate on any images, or experiences. They are just experiences. Everything that occurs during the meditation is all good. It is all part of this mysterious alchemy of healing.

THE WEAVER

"Hungering, hungering, hungering, for primal energies and Nature's dauntlessness."

—Walt Whitman, Leaves of Grass.

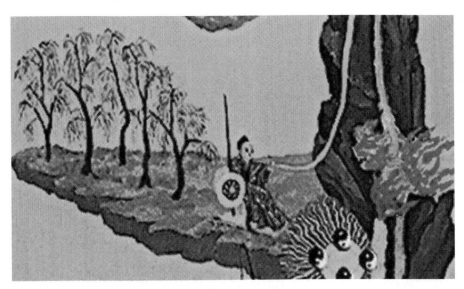

Descending deeper into the inner landscape painting we see the spleen depicted as the weaver—moonfaced, tranquility in repose, spinning a wheel of silk bundles. She is an iconic figure, sedate and meditative in her long flowing golden silk robe. The weaver is, of course, a symbol—the entity that pulls in the strands of nourishment and energy (the grain Qi) from the raw bulk of ingested foods as she sits upon a green grotto of willow trees, the Liver. It is a stroke of pure genius to place the weaver and the willow grove together, as the spleen and liver overlap each other at the midsection of the body. As the spleen pulls in the strands of nutrients, the arboreal liver function acts similarly to an Amazonian rainforests—dispersing and attenuating the energetic fluidity in the body. Moreover, in an insightful graphic illustration, one sees the weaver seated squarely on top of a ledge jutting out of the rocky vertebra column. This indicates the liver's function as a support for the spleen's digestive process. Accordingly, the creator of this image encapsulates the entire theory of TCM within the landscape; the axiom that a picture is worth a thousand words becomes resoundingly clear.

Personified as the weaver, the spleen becomes synonymous with the psychological attributes of patience and endurance. It should be noted that the antitheses of these qualities are the pathological emotions of apprehension, anxiety and lethargy. We can therefore deduce that the spleen is responsible for self-healing. This spontaneous healing power rests squarely on the shoulders of the weaver, the spleen. Herein is the divergence between Chinese Medicine and western scientific medical theory.

Western medical science seldom attributes psychological factors to the internal organs; it is incomprehensible to attribute lethargy to a weakened spleen otherwise known as hypo-splenic metabolism in medical terminology. Not so for TCM doctors, they deduced from clinical experience that emotions and the mind are intrinsically interwoven with the physical organs of the body. The Chinese delineated in great detail the connection between mind and body two thousand years ago in the canonical text, *The Yellow Emperor's Treatise on Inner Medicine*. Consequently, the Inner Landscape is a pictorial illustration of the text, and much more; encrypted in the image is condensed the entire Taoist inner alchemical cultivation as well. Ah, but alas, here lies the rub, the image is without textual explanation and therefore presumes the presence of a competent teacher to reveal its inner secret to a novice. The image serves as a means to safeguard the secret that is intended for initiates only and therefore, avoids exploitation by unscrupulous charlatans.

Unfortunately, oral transmission from master to disciple can be easily broken; wars, famine, personal misfortunes and political persecution have severed many ancient lineages. In the latest episode of dissolution in China, the Cultural Revolution literally vanquished a whole generation of old masters with one gigantic stroke; their wisdom and knowledge will be buried with them forever. Fortunately, a few escaped to the West and were able to pass on their insights and humanity's treasure to the next generation.

Thus the Inner Landscape image serves as a compressed encyclopedic training manual for both TCM students as well as a deeper layer of encoded instruction for inner alchemical cultivation. To fully delineate and decode the complete image is way beyond the nature and scope of this book, requiring minimally a book of its own. Readers interested in researching the Inner Landscape further should seek out an alchemist to guide them further into the depths of this most profound and enigmatic picture book of immortality. I have included the Inner Landscape both as a cursory introduction to TCM as well as a resource for the readers. Though the Inner Landscape is fascinating, we must now leave the painting and return to our topic of healing cancer.

The Ockham's razor of cancer therapy cuts to the quick of cancer treatment in TCM: Healing cancer relies on the self-healing power of the patient. Accordingly, the spleen's capacity to absorb nutrients and provide nourishment is at the center stage of cancer healing. The following chapter of a two hundred-year-old clinical cancer healing project in China will demonstrate quite comprehensively this hypothesis.

THE WATER WHEEL OF LIFE

In the valley at the base of the Sacred Mountain, we encounter a pair of chubby, cherubic prepubescent youngsters treading gleefully atop an antique water-wheel, an agrarian high-tech invention enabling the reversal of a stream's current and used to irrigate the rice paddies located above. The two round forms with their rotary function, an astute reader will guess no doubt its metaphoric stand-in: the testes in the male or the ovaries in the female.

In the science of embryology, the male testes in embryo are retained inside the fetus's abdominal cavity. As the embryo develops, they descend down through the oblique passage of the inguinal canal and then through the lower abdominal wall. This is the opening through which the testes descend to the scrotum. Therefore, in essence, the testes and ovaries resemble each other, and both store the germinal seeds of life. Given that sperm require a temperature cooler than 98.6°F to survive and thrive, it thus necessitates the scrotum hang outside the body cavity. For the female, however, the ovaries need to remain inside the body in order for the egg, once emitted by the ovary, to swim across the body fluid to the fallopian tube—a re-enactment of the primal sexual dance of fish spawning.

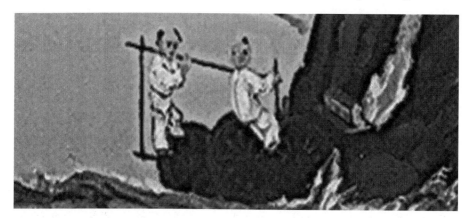

Gleaning from the functions of our reproductive system, we can deduce that evolutionarily our most ancient organs are the testes and ovaries. Sperm still swim upstream to impregnate the egg that floats in the fluid of the female's inner ocean. Being human, rather than fish or amphibians, we carry the ocean within us. However our mating dance still resembles the fluidic grace of beluga whales undulating in the primal sea and within this secret sanctum rests one of the oldest instinctive behaviors. The origins of sex can be traced back to the first blind deep-sea creatures attracted to one another by smell and movement. Notwithstanding, sex is the quintessential primary factor needed for survival, thus generating competition amongst most species on Earth. For homo sapiens, (Latin for: humanly wise) sex is, nevertheless, caged by the rigid Judeo-Christian culture, and other religious, social and moral codes—stray from these norms, and you risk the full wrath of societal constraints. History is strewn with tragic figures of sexual deviation—considered miscreants destined for prosecution, execution and incineration for nothing more than behaviors that stray from expected conduct.

Fortunately, in Taoist alchemical practice, there are no such prohibitions or inhibitions. The natural cycle of life must include sex and sexuality; it is part of the whole of being human. The ubiquitous Confucius argued that drink, food, and sex are fundamental needs of human nature. Nonetheless, there is a certain celibate Taoist monastic order that lives a life of austerity from the senses and hence, sexual cravings are rejected as unwholesome and a carnal entrapment. Moreover, this group of hyper-male renunciates have become obsessed with sperm due to their belief that men just like women have only a limited quantity of seed and once this store is completely depleted death will follow. However if one abstains from sex, the drainage of one's sperm ceases and the life force is retained. As this notion proliferated, variants of practices for the householder developed. Novices are taught to press against the sperm duct in order to block the flow of ejaculation during sexual intercourse. As was mentioned earlier, this manipulation has the grave unintended consequence of prostatitis (an inflammation of the prostate). Therefore, it would seem that this technique is a result of a misinterpretation of the reversal of sexual flow as it relates to the rejuvenation process as depicted in the Inner Landscape painting.

As illustrated, the outflow of fluid from deep inside the subterranean stream drains into the sea and is analogous to the process of male ejaculation—the outpouring of seminal liquid to impregnate the egg inside the woman's womb, or inner ocean and thus re-enacting the primal spawning ritual. In Taoist texts, it is often said that by allowing the outflow of orgasmic ejaculation life will be created, but reversing the process will lead to immortality. Therefore, in light of this image, wholeness and healing perhaps depend upon reversing, retaining and storing the sexual energy either for the spiritual purpose of enlightenment, or in the case of this book's premise, to heal sickness. Hence, the pair of cherubic undying children churn back the drainage of one's seminal fluid enacting the metaphor for the alchemical yoga of regeneration. Rather than creating a new life, one turns this generative life-stream back to oneself and gives birth to one's own immortal child.

The legendary immortal Lu Dong Bing (500 AD) is said to have failed several time in having spontaneous seminal emission (wet dreams), and only after a long and arduous esoteric progression was he able to achieve immortality. A tall tale perhaps but to Taoist initiates they hold this account to be true and real. In an early archaic form of Tibetan tantric ritual, the disciples were fed a most bizarre concoction composed of breast milk, mead, menstrual blood, and seminal fluid. Similarly, Taoists are obsessed with sexual secretions, or Jing, 精; they regard it as the most precious treasure of life and the liquid state of condensed life force. When Jing is distilled through the esoteric yoga of Qigong, the arcane movements and breathing practices transmogrifies one's Jing into the higher permeable gaseous state of Qi, 气. In the view of the organic alchemist, our body is composed of a singular unifying life-force differentiated into variegated states:

First: Luminous Bio-electro-magnetic State, Shen, 神, spirit or numen, the field of consciousness and all mental processes.

Second: Gaseous State, Qi, the all-pervasive energy and force that is required for all biological activity.

Third: Liquid State, Jing, sexual fluids and endocrine hormones.

Taoist genesis describes the creation of the universe as a spontaneous combustion arising out of emptiness or the void; this is the singular occurrence from which Shen originates. Out of the vacuum of emptiness, the field of consciousness, Shen, is born. From this first stage of a formless numinous field, a part becomes heavy and degrades into Qi—the second stage and gaseous state of energy. From Qi, the life force condenses further, acquiring viscosity and finally turns into Jing, the third stage and state of liquid form. It is from this tertiary phase that this liquid spirals downward to form corporeal solids of bones, muscles, tendons, vascular system etc. and produces a materialized being. Within this cosmic paradigm, the goal of Taoist alchemical cultivation is to reverse this downward degenerative flow and return the seminal Jing back to Qi and by an upward regenerative flow to restore the Qi back to the numinous Shen. Hence at the pinnacle of Taoist achievement, one returns to the pristine original state of emptiness. Lao Tzu, the Socrates of the Chinese people, wrote in his famous book, Tao Te Ching, "The function of all things lies within their capacity to be empty. Think of a bowl, its real use is when it is empty so that we can pour food into it. Think of the hub of a wheel, its use is in its spaciousness allowing the spokes to converge and join at the center. And finally, in one's dwelling, is it not space that makes one's living quarter roomy and functional?"

This merging of consciousness with vast emptiness is analogous to the reversal of genesis. Hence, generations of Taoists have meditated in utter stillness, in deep ecstasy. The alchemist lives this reverse voyage in meditation in order to be transformed; one's existence is wholly other, no longer mortal but not quite immortal yet.

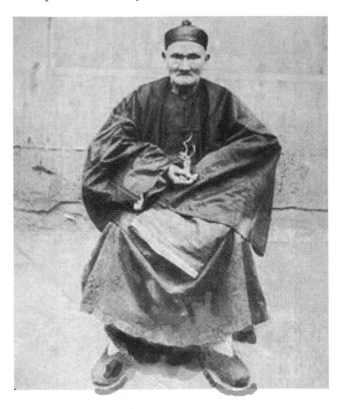

A MODERN DAY 250 YEAR-OLD TAOIST

In recent times, in the 1930s at the foothills of Szechuan, a wizen Taoist, Li Qīngyún,　李清雲, (1677-1933) was discovered by the Warlord Yang Seng. Li was a herbalist who allegedly lived to be over 256 years old. When he was interviewed and pressed for his true age, Li maintained that he was born in 1677. My late Taoist master, H.K. Gu served as a young lieutenant under the Warlord Yang Sheng and was invited to a banquet in Li's honor. Later on, lieutenant Gu consulted with Li who bestowed to him his herbal formula for longevity, as well as several qigong forms. Li's claim of longevity could not be verified by historical documentation or official records of imperial post during the Manchu dynasty. However, he was allegedly awarded a commendation for his supreme skill as a herbalist (1777). Nevertheless, if one examines his one existing portrait (a photograph taken by

Yang Seng), his physique and mental acuity appear to be respectively vital and alert. On closer inspection, he maintained the antiquated custom of growing his nails extremely long resembling windblown branches spiraling upward. Quite tragically, the two-hundred-fifty year-old man died within a year after his exposure. No doubt the excessive stress of adoration, press interviews and dinner banquets took their toll. During one of the interviews, Li revealed quite openly his longevity secret: Meditation, vegetarianism and special herbal supplements. At my late master's ninetieth birthday celebration, Gu revealed Li's secret formula of Longevity Tea: Goji Berry juice. Goji Berry (also known as Wolf Berry in the West) has an effect of rejuvenating one's sexual libido. Furthermore, Gu claimed that the essence of Li's long life was keeping an open spirit, joyous living and forgetfulness. Or as my ninety-two year-old mother would say, "Why bother remembering the bad stuff of life?!" So true.

As part of the training in Taoist Inner Alchemy in the tradition of the Complete Perfection School of the Dragon Gate, there is a form of meditation that is both formless and transformative. I was initiated into this inner sanctum of Alchemy and its initiates are guided by a poetic verse, *Song of the Clear Sky*, written by the great Taoist alchemical master, Qiu Chuji, (1148–1227 AD). This epoch was historically a most violent and chaotic time in China with the impending invasion of the Mongolian army. Qiu Chuji was invited by Genghis Khan to visit him in eastern Mongolia. Genghis Khan requested Qiu's help in his search for immortality and longevity (as most tyrants and conquerors seem to desire). But the Taoist master told him that in all honesty there was no secret of immortality and no elixir. The only way to live a long healthy life is to cultivate loving kindness. This must have taken some guts to preach to a blood thirsty Genghis who sacked and massacred whole cities and towns that dared to resist.

According to legend, Qiu did perform a minor miracle for the Kahn by turning lead into gold in order to validate his mastery in alchemy. Henceforth, Genghis granted to Qiu's followers immunity from his army by giving Qiu a copper talisman and iron scroll/picture as proof. Any person who carries such copies of talisman or hangs them on their gate would be saved. Naturally, Qiu's Taoist Dragon Gate sect became widely popular and acquired masses of followers. Whether this account is historically accurate or not is beside the point; it illustrates how one person with a deep sense of equanimity and wisdom can save a multitude of lives from one act of kindness. Qiu's journey to the West concluded when he finally caught up with the Kahn in the Hindu Kush. No doubt his travels must have been filled with perils and obstacles but in doing so, Qiu laid a vast foundation for later generations of alchemists. The poem below is a distillation of a lifetime's meditational cultivation and serves as a luminous guide for inner alchemists and their search for enlightenment.

These days, the modern-day spiritual *gurus* of the media dispense their words of wisdom to the masses seated beside famous celebrity TV talkshow hosts and discuss the virtue and "power of NOW" or they power walk with their thousand dollar pair of ruby-red designer snickers. Their audience is hardly able to afford to pay rent or medical bills. At the end of the day barely able to keep their heads above water, they find themselves falling into a stupor in front of a flickering TV screen with a crumpled beer can in hand. So, in desperate attempts toward a spiritual redemption, most seek an easy way out through charms, mantras, higher spiritual teachings and magic; in belief that these may bestow a reliable cure for life's ills. They search for a method, an unvanquishable secret to unleash them, but alas their hopes hang by a single breathtaking thread. A conquering spirit is perhaps the antidote to this spiritual materialism and the halo effect's delusion. What is required is a return to the Self, as a man or woman, in one's ordinary unfabricated state of Being. And that is enough. What follows below is an ancient teaching to guide one toward Self-discovery. Only a wise person will recognize the truth of its profound simplicity and will try to follow it. Whereas fools would surely laugh and belittle it as mere mumbo-jumbo. But for most, they will slough through the language as if hearing a strange foreign tongue.

These early esoteric texts can be somewhat obtuse, in their use of arcane metaphors: the iron flute, the Jade Princeling child riding backward, the string-less Stellar Zither…. However, if you possess the spirit of a diamond miner, you can dig deep into the heart of the shamanic psyche, and possibly find a means to remedy your sickness and despair. Like a man who stands chin-deep in a pool of water and all the while dying of thirst, to my utter astonishment, I discovered this means has always been available. Hence, a word from the wise: "Consistently turn your gaze back to its origin." As to what this really means, practice the meditation of the Clear Sky below, and you shall find out.

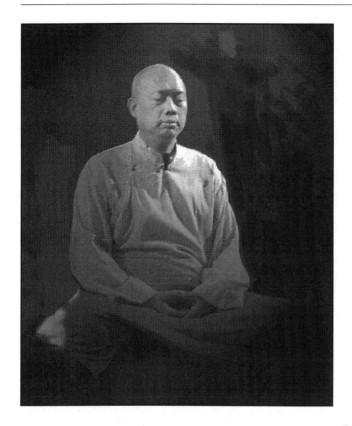

SONG OF QINGTIAN

Clear azure sky

nothing should arise

not even a floating cloud obscures

Arousal clouds the cerulean sky

veiling the myriad phenomenon

The ten thousand things in their evanescence

suppress the hundred deviants

Their radiant luminosity dimmed

as the shadowy sinister Mara surges

During my initial opening

heaven and earth became lucid and clear

O how the ten thousand families and thousand folk

sing out the Hoshana of Supreme Peace

In the moment when a strand of darkened cloud arises

the nine orifices, hundred bones all churn and fret without end

Henceforth strengthen the teachings of Prajna

like a fierce gust of strong wind

May the three realms, ten directions

be thus buffeted and cleansed thoroughly

As clouds disperse

the clear spacious emptiness emerges

and the self-nature of un-fabricated reality is suddenly realized

Spontaneously the full moon appears over house after house in an unending lineage

Only then could one dare to play the reedy flute under the clear moonlight

A single note pierces and shakes even to the world's end

It even awakens the Eastern Jade princeling Child

As he straddles the white musk deer backward, like a drunkard

It gallops as quick as a shooting star

The penetrating ecstatic sound is unlike any ordinary pleasure

Ah t'is not quite the tune of the Zither

Not quite the Horn

The three feet ancient Zither, Yuan Hu,

encompasses the twelve musical tones and star constellations

Throughout the three kalpas the primordial chaos is cut

The crisp resonance akin to the swirling sound of jade beads falling

silences the internal dialogue

A pristine lightness permeates and overflows in my heart

Henceforth having awakened to Oneness

demons and devas empower me

Diving into the underworld and soaring to heaven

I transcend the present and past

Traversing the ten directions, sideways or upward

Abiding in suchness of being

Free of all hindrances and compulsion

Mind free of lust for fame

Body free of all besmirchment

Thus in languor

I sing the song of powdery white snow

sloshing in my immortal gourd

In quiescence I tune the hermitical melody of Sunny Spring

Throughout my long lineage, this song has always spontaneously arisen

O blow upon an iron flute without holes

Ah pluck the stringless lute

How startling to have wakened

from this floating dream of life

Day and night the chant of penetrating clarity

fills and echoes in my celestial cavern

translated by Sat Hon, July 2014

At the heart of alchemical meditation is a non-willful way of being. In other words, if you meditate with the intention to become calm, or to relax or even to search for enlightenment, awakening or release, then even these seemly "good" intentions are just more clouds in your clear sky/consciousness. Once thoughts, intentions or subliminal urges arise, the original clarity of your self-nature is obscured; everything is hidden and you are lost. Hence, even the thought of "being here now" is another form of cloudiness. As my late Master Nan once said, "The very first instant of sitting down to meditate is the best chance to be under a clear sky/consciousness. Right then, you are not yet concerned with practicing stillness, dispersing thoughts or even contemplating the divine through visualization. You just sit and that's it. But alas, our monkey mind refuses to accept such simplicity and is compelled to search and struggle for enlightenment. Our deluded minds are convinced that tremendous effort is the only way to awaken and that it must be earned in order to be real. But how can anything that is learned or cultivated be abiding? The clear blue sky is self-abiding clarity without taint of self-conscious deliberation. When you are finally emptied of deliberation, spontaneously the clear sky appears then everything opens and the whole universe lay open in the palm of your hand just like a lotus blossom." Ah, that simple. Perchance, the Tao in its great simplicity is so easily overlooked and generations upon generations of practitioners fall into the abyss of duplicity, delusion and degeneration.

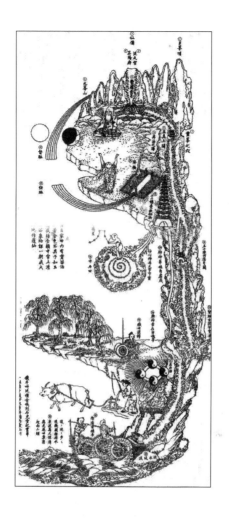

CHAPTER EIGHT: A TWO HUNDRED YEAR CANCER STUDY

A CHINESE LOVE STORY

The story begins with a humble young servant smuggling food to her lover (an ex-mendicant monk) who will later join the revolution to overthrow the Mongols. On this morning, she shivers in the cold bleak Szechuan winter and weeps silently while reaching into her bosom (the only place where the guards will not dare to search). She produces a burning loaf of bread that has scalded her skin forming ugly red blisters. This single act of love sparks enormous consequences: the defeat of the Mongolian invaders resulting in the founding of an empire and tragically, a seed of cancer for the future queen. For the ex-monk is destined to become the emperor of China.

Three decades later, on a bright spring day, the emperor summoned the imperial physician. The queen had developed an open sore on her breast. Initially, various herbs and ointments were prescribed, but they failed and the sores multiplied. Only then did the royal physician's heart sink. He realized that the queen had a rare pathology, a type of ossified rocklike tumor (breast cancer) that could be traced back to the intense burn from the scalding bread. To constrain the cancer's incessant growth, the physician prescribed shark's gall bladder, a highly caustic digestive juice that corrodes the stomach lining. This negative side effect caused the queen to lose her appetite and her appearance started to resemble that of an ancient gnarled cypress.

Treating the queen's cancer was paramount for the royal physician as the Emperor was already in a helpless rage over the decline of his beloved queen. In his grief, he had already executed several of the court physician's predecessors. Subsequently, if he could save the queen's life, he would also rescue his own. "Physician, heal thyself" in this instance became quite literal.

A RAY OF HOPE

The imperial physician walked past a prisoner with a robust, round face wearing a rough, sackcloth vest—a designation of his impending death. The bullock cart rumbled along the ancient road delivering the man to the marketplace to be publicly executed; the physician wondered whether his crime was of passion, murder, greed or robbery. The executioner stood beside him cradling a long curved scimitar—no doubt the prisoner's family bribed him handsomely to behead him with one merciful stroke. The caged man gazed down at him with a hunger to live; he pleaded, sighed and crumbled to the floor. As the physician passed the prisoner on his way to the Royal Medical College, he contemplated this tragic waste of a man in the prime of his life.

He, himself, the royal court physician, had failed utterly in healing the queen's cancer. Not being an expert in this disease, he felt that he was a mere hack, learned in several classical texts in medicine with a hundred or so memorized herbal formulas. What is the saying? 'Only heal sickness that is curable, and avoid the one that is incurable.' The queen's cancer is terminal yet the royal command forced him to treat an incurable disease. His reflection shone in the puddles left over from last night's rainstorm as his sandals indented deeply into the soggy mud. He had utterly failed; the cancer resurfaced with clusters of dark brown, grape-sized tumors encroaching distinctly over her entire body. The cancer was taking over and would eventually replace the healthy tissues of her body with itself. The terminal stage was approaching and it seemed that whatever herbs: shark's gallbladder, ginseng, rishi mushroom; all were ineffective against the cancer's merciless progression.

Engrossed in contemplation of his dilemma, unknowingly, the famous royal court physician reached the marketplace; the crowd parted for the queen's favorite personal doctor. There tied to a wooden pole was the prisoner eating his last meal: a bowl of rice with a heaping stack of fried dumplings. The court physician laughed hysterically at this ludicrous scene. He thought *at least this man will not die hungry.* But then he grew somber and thought, "Am I not also only giving palliative care to the queen?" He drifted toward the prisoner unaware, like a moth being drawn by a flame of agony and terror. He instinctively wanted to offer the poor chap some peace, absolution, and perhaps a ray of hope.

When the guards roughly shoved him away from the prisoner, a sudden flash of inspiration flared like a beacon in him, "Why not use death row inmates as subjects for cancer research and experiments?" By creating known contributing factors such as mental and physical stress, trauma, toxic herbs and the most crucial ingredient of all, starvation, he could artificially induce cancer. By systematically depleting the body's immune system to defend the disease, there is a high probability that most of the inmates will develop tumors, and a small percentage will develop cancer. "A diabolical experiment," he reflected, "But at least it will give them a fighting chance. If they survive, the emperor would surely give them back their lives and freedom."

"Stop the execution!" he yelled out. "The queen needs this man as her medicine." The residing official recognized the court physician, a powerful man with high connections. So the execution was stayed. The doomed prisoner was unbound and he ran to kowtow at the physician's feet. The physician pulled the man to his feet and whispered, "Ah, Sir, you might just save both of our lives."

The Cancer Experiment

Clinical cancer trials may strike us with awe, inspiration, fear, attraction or repulsion. Cancer invades the human body, the supreme treasured entity that is both fragile and irreplaceable. Cancer research reveals the detours, the dead ends and more recently the right paths toward healing this insidious disease. Ancient healers investigated by trial and error, exposing their folly mistaking cancer as either a type of infection, or a sort of bacterial fungi radiating from a nucleus in ever expanding growth. These misconceptions of cancer led to one of the most erroneous medical procedures in the West, radical surgery—the practice of removing the tumors and healthy neighboring tissues. Considering the recent perception of cancer as a genetic disease and not an infection or fungal growth, reveals that the wrong narrative of the disease can lead to fatal mistakes in treatment.

Such errors fortunately did not occur in the ancient Chinese understanding of cancer. In TCM, cancer had a different narrative based on the whole picture of illness. Illness at its core is a stagnation of one's energy and humors; at the same time it prompts examination of the spirit, the mind.

In following a two hundred-year-old cancer trial, we see the passion of physicians and the bravery of common people in a battle of insurmountable odds. We witness how these people live and how they die. At the center of the narrative, there is always a hero versus a villain, and at the fulcrum, a trial.

How does the physician disentangle the mystery of cancer's myriad symptoms? What is this disease? How does the physician set up the conditions to induce the occurrence of cancer in his subjects? Even now with modern 21st century medical advances, it is still extremely hard to induce cancer in animals. He was compelled by the king's command to accomplish the set-up, the solution and result in relatively short order to save or at least extend the queen's life and therefore, his own. This was the challenge the imperial doctor faced as he began his clinical trials on the death row inmates.

THE SET UP

Four hundred years ago, 1600 A.D., if you were sick you would have a much better chance of being cured in China than anywhere else in the world. In England, Queen Elizabeth I was treated with bloodletting to expunge the evil from her body. However, the poison came from a white power made with lead that she used as a cosmetic. When most of the world was in the dark ages of medicine, Chinese medicinal treatment, in contrast, was a guiding light with its knowledge of clearing stagnated energy.

In setting up his clinical experiment, the physician needed a population of subjects with the disease and a control group to compare the effectiveness of the treatment. Herein lies the dilemma for the royal physician, cancer in those times was a rare disease and in his lifetime, he had only seen a handful of cancer patients. Furthermore, he desperately required a model of the disease.

Since Chinese is a language based on pictures, icons, symbols and metaphors, the very word, *Amg*, depicts a rocklike aggregate of tumors piled into a mound. The Chinese character, *Amg*, can be traced back to Neolithic origins. The image that comes to mind is that of a pile of rocks stacked up as an offering to the Gods at the highest pass. How apropos is this offering of sickness and plague to the gods?

In TCM theory, differential diagnosis is based on four cardinal signs: pulse, tongue coloration, physical symptoms and mental state. For example, a middle-aged man comes in with a raging headache after a night of drinking and carousing. He will most likely be diagnosed as being excessively Yin due to the infiltration of pathological wind damage. To a novice, this will sound like Greek! However, to a Chinese physician steeped in a cultural milieu where metaphor, analogy and symbolism are commonplace and the Emperor *is* the Son of Heaven seated on a dragon throne; the physician will be able to use this symbolic diagnoses to prescribe and concoct an herbal formula to combat the excessive Yin (or, state of depletion). A common herbal formula for a hangover is Ginger broth with a dash of honey to warm the body.

Cancer with its rock-hard carcinoma is given the metaphor of a fossilized rock, a biological calcification of the life force. Cancer epitomizes excessive Yang with its aggressive life force. It is the final crystallization of pathological energy—a masterless wandering ronin that hardens within the stagnant network of energy channels (the meridians). Subsequently Cancer manifests in diverse symptoms and behavior. Some tumors are inherently dormant like a silent stone Buddha, and others proliferate dividing and multiplying like bamboo shoots. To address the inherent diversity of various types of cancer, the royal physician came up with an ingenious method to induce the disease: stress.

In his many years of clinical practice, he observed a direct correlation between the onset of serious illness following extremely stressful situations. Without modern knowledge regarding stress and its effect on the adrenal glands and such, he was able to deduce this trigger from direct clinical observation: extreme stress followed by illness. From the TCM perspective, the external pathogens require an internal pathogenic environment (a depleted immune system) in order for the diseases to take root. Subsequently, in his very first clinical trial, he set up stressful situations for the death row inmates by requiring them to memorize randomly chosen passages; failure to perform would be treated with a harsh whipping and other punishments. The modern reader might shudder at such outright cruelty and judge these human experiments as unethical, but from the perspective of a death row inmate at least there was a glimmer of hope for life and freedom.

As anticipated, after half a year of such strain, various forms of disease manifested. A majority exhibited psychological symptoms but no cancer. Cancer as we now know is due to cellular mutation and required an extended period for development. Without such knowledge, our imperial physician had to inject into the stress some other element to induce the occurrence of cancer. Fortunately, in TCM pathology, the spleen is the dominant organ for spontaneous healing and regeneration. Accordingly, the physician ordered the prison guards to decrease the prisoner's food intake by 50% and within months, tumors started to emerge like grapes in many older female inmates.

Finally, the lethal combination of stress plus malnourishment created the conditions for the development of the dreaded disease.

Having succeeded in creating a small population of cancer patients, the physician started to concoct herbal formulas to cure them. The obvious choice is to reverse the condition by removing the stress and feeding nutritional food. However, once cancer had taken root, it cannot be reversed by those measures alone. Meanwhile, the queen's cancer was still getting worse. The ingestion of the Shark's Gall Bladder had slowed the growth of the tumors, but at the same time, its corrosive juice had also destroyed her stomach lining and consequently, her appetite. The queen was growing thinner and thinner every day. The emperor had become desperate to find a cure and summoned the physician for news of his findings. So far, no such remedy was found.

Harkening back to his days as a disciple with his master, the royal physician recollected his master saying, "Heal a dead horse like a live one." Through this arcane saying, the teacher was guiding the young novice to deal with the symptoms of the sickness, and steering him to avoid deduction of the pathology. Armed with this revelation, the royal physician treated the queen's nausea with an herbal broth composed mainly of sweet fruity hawthorn berries and the blood enriching Goji berries in bone marrow broth. At least this kept the queen from losing weight.

Subsequently, the physician prescribed the same herbal remedy to his cancer subjects and to his astonishment some of the tumors in several cancer patients started to disappear. Unfortunately, however, the cancer took a firm hold on a majority of the subjects.

Parallel to modern cancer researchers who inject an array chemicals and drugs into tubes of cancer cells, the physician searched far and wide for effective herbal ingredients: scorpions, shark's fin, lizard, a thousand herbal roots, flowers, fruit, bark and grasses. In desperation, he even tried the highly toxic alchemical agent, mercury with lethal results. None had given him the panacea that he fervently needed. After almost ten years, the queen finally succumbed to her breast cancer and died. On her deathbed, she held the emperor's hand and bid him not to punish the court physician. She asked that he support the continuation of his cancer research so that a cure could be found. At her behest the Ming emperor consented. It was fortunate indeed for the court physician, in anticipation of the emperor's wrath, he had already written his final will and testament having failed to find a cure for the queen.

The emperor kept his promise, but as he could not stand the sight of the man who failed to save his wife, he instead banished him to the nether regions of China. The death row inmates were all set free. However, during the ten-year-long cancer trial all but a few of the inmates survived, eventually earning their freedom. The court physician quite astutely observed one last important occurrence: After being freed, some of the prisoners' cancer spontaneously vanished. It seemed as though the joy of freedom and reunion with their families was the most potent cancer remedy.

Even during his exile in southern China, so far from the capital, the ex-court physician continued his research and generations after him continued his work for two hundred years. From this dedicated family of healers, a new modality of healing took shape: 70% nourishment and 30% medicine. The balance between nourishment and medicine became the de-facto gold standard for all Chinese herbal formulas, acupuncture treatments and qigong routines.

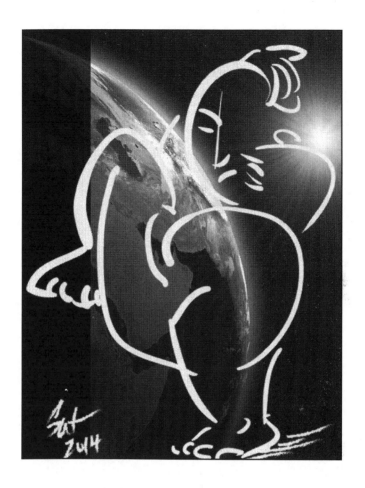

Chapter Nine: The Healing Dance of the Cosmos

"I have created the Healing Walk Qigong to combat the onslaught of my own incurable metastatic carcinoma..."

—Gou Lin

Many aspects of healing have no name, and many cures, even if they have a name, have never been fully delineated. The term Complementary Healing Art—is a variant of alternative healing but hardly identical to it. It often goes by the more common acronym, CHA .

Complementary Healing (as distinct from alternative healing) is one of the most intricate and obtuse aspects of healing; however, there are reasons why CHA, in particular, has so far rarely been discussed. It is not the typical allopathic mode of fighting disease, if there be any such. Undeniably, the essence of complementary healing is its inclusiveness of the spontaneous self-healing power. It includes as well the use of movement, Qigong and the ever evanescence human spirit. Hence, CHA is esoteric—somewhat of an exclusive domain for a few privileged vanguards of alternative medicine. I am lucky to be amongst them having been trained in both Traditional Chinese medicine and Qigong.

Since this book serves as a guide to the Complementary approach toward healing cancer, it is the perfect place to begin our journey to investigate the healing dance of qigong. The essence of qigong is the breath, after all, the very word, Qi, literally means breath or air. Therefore, the healing walk is mindful breathing as one walks. It is a way to relax the mind and diminish the stresses of coping with cancer. The alchemy of healing relies on these four components: breath, body, mind and spirit. (For a video demonstration of this walk, please go to the website: www.qigongtherapy.com)

The breath is the quintessential process that allows the healing process to take place. In Taoist healing, breath encompasses not only physical respiration, but also the subtle flow of inner Qi that circulates within. This deep Qi is moreover the cosmic breath that permeates everywhere and everything. This all-pervasive understanding of the breath often bewilders many novices of qigong, and even more so cancer patients burdened with the stress of an uncertain future. Even so, the heart of Taoist healing weaves the four components (breath, body, mind and spirit) into one unified life force to help us battle the spread of cancer as well as the secondary effects frequently experienced from standard cancer treatments.

How do these qigong breaths interact with each other? From the internal alchemist's perspective, as one inhales and draws the air down into the lungs, simultaneously one's inner Qi rises up to meet the external breath. A swirling motion is usually described as the process of their interaction. The inner Qi acquires nutrients from the outer breath and then descends to the abdominal region during exhalation. In addition, subterranean channels within our body link our organs, muscles and brain. These channels flow like underground streams and the inner Qi moves in a circadian rhythm according to a designated schedule. The accompanying chart shows the time schedule of the ebb and flow of Qi in the channels.

Imagine each organ as series of cataracts facilitating the descent of a high mountain stream. As the water tumbles from one organ to another, the stream brings with it nutrients and thus nourishes that particular organ. Positioned at the highest plateau are the lungs which are energetically connected to the colon. The lungs are more than just an apparatus for breathing. In TCM, the lungs also guard and defend the body against marauding invaders and microbial infections as they are in direct contact with the external environment through the process of respiration. No wonder, the lungs are considered a second layer of skin, but internally, the lungs resemble a porous wet sponge flooded with blood and blood vessels.

ORGAN	TIME	FN/MOTION	PATHOLOGY
Lungs	3-5 am	immune defense, descending Qi downward	cough, asthma, immune weakness, COPD, clinical depression
Colon	5-7 am	elimination	constipation, indecisiveness
Stomach	7-9 am	digestion	acid reflux, ulcer, difficulty in swallowing
Spleen/ pancreas	9-11 am	transport nutrient upward, transform food into nourishing Qi, purge downward waste	anorexia, slow healing, excessive anxiety
Heart	11-1 pm	warmth, consciousness, awareness, mental thoughts, upward thrust of Qi	mental disorder, psychosis, insomnia, mental retardation, manic
Small Intestine	1-3 pm	absorption of nutrient	high fever, indecision, inability to digest food

ORGAN	TIME	FN/MOTION	PATHOLOGY
Bladder	3-5 pm	dispersal of urine, downward flow	UTI, incontinent, frequent urination, tension back headaches
Kidneys	5-7 pm	store sexual essence, control body liquid, upward thrust of Qi	impotence, infertility, chronic fatigue, lack of libido
Pericardium	7-9 pm	heart, circulation, emotion	arrhythmia, heart diseases, coronary blockage, insomnia
Triple Warmer	9-11 pm	disseminate nutrients and Qi to belly, torso & chest	immune deficiency, Hashimoto, hyperthyroidism, flu, high fever
Gall Bladder	11-1 am	will, mental acuity, emotional stability	hyper-vigilance, indigestion oily food, timidity
Liver	1-3 am	store blood, smooth Qi flow	explosive rage, Parkinson, MS, spontaneous movement

Following the stream, it cascades down to the spleen which connects energetically to the stomach. As we have already learned from the previous chapter, the spleen is the organ for spontaneous healing and rejuvenation as well as the organ responsible for absorbing nutrients. Since it absorbs food, it thus provides the materials for mending and healing the body from the ravages of disease.

Continuing its downward flow, the mountain rivulet seeps down to the heart which serves not only as a physical pump for the blood, but is also the seat of consciousness. How one deciphers this statement is up to you. However, within Chinese culture, it is understood that one feels and thinks with the heart. Thus, even within popular "foodie" culture, the two compound words of "dim" "sum," translate as a little bit of heart's delight. In TCM, the heart functions also as a warming agent for the circulation.

In its relentless downward flow, the stream falls from the heart into the lower region of the kidneys. Here the metaphorical conception of the kidneys being organs of sexuality, the retainer of one's procreative essence, (as opposed to being solely organs of blood filtration) can easily overwhelm the uninitiated. The shape of the kidney resembles in its outline a fetus in fetal position in the womb and additionally the kidney also retains the elemental assignation of water. Ancient alchemists realized that the ocean is the mother from which all life originated and sexuality harkens back to the mating of fish. A white fish and black fish swirl around and around in a spawning frenzy to become the icon for the ancient symbol, Taiji. Therefore, the two kidneys are metaphorically conceived as the two fecund fishes; in the heat of passion, sexual fluid is secreted from the kidneys down to one's sex organ.

Since the Chinese maintain that the kidney is a watery organ, it therefore stores the seminal creative fluid, (the Jing). Interestingly, they also happen to be the organs that grow in the very initial embryonic gestation of a fetus. And in astute observation of post-coital interaction, most men would in general feel a slight soreness in their lower back and this leads to the deduction that the kidneys are being drained. For a thousand years, Cantonese dietary nutrition is fixated on nourishing these organs with Goji berry, Angelica or *Dong Gui*, and ingesting pig's kidney to deal with a host of watery issues such as incontinence, impotence, or lack of sexual desire. And in Qigong, the waist rotation is solely done to warm up the kidneys. Not only do the kidneys store the seminal fluid, or ovarian hormone for women, they also store the potential pre-natal life force. This pre-natal force could be equated with how many times a rechargeable battery can be recharged. As we age, we no longer restore our energy as fast as when we were young and this is viewed as a sign of the depletion or in other words the drainage of the pre-natal life force. When the kidneys are weak, so is the bone marrow and CSF of the brain and thus this leads to Osteoporosis and various age related mental illness. Thus, it is often said that the practice of qigong is solely to nourish the kidneys in order to keep this degeneration to a minimum.

Once the stream has reached the nadir, its water starts to evaporate and rise up toward the liver. The liver with its auxiliary organ, the gallbladder, absorbs the water and in turn emits moisture through its leaves thus permeating the entire body with moisture. When the liver (the treelike organ) becomes too dry, the liver's wild fire burns and causes uncontrollable rage in us. Maybe that is why we call a raging person livid with anger, a state of such rage that their blood turned dark purple due to the momentary constriction of blood vessels in their face and the liver's release of the enzyme, Glycogen, into the blood stream.

In summary, our being is nourished by Qi, an inner life stream that tumbles from organ to organ and in turn serves us by keeping our organ functions working smoothly. Sickness occurs when the stream stagnates, becoming a waterway choked with weeds or debris. From a stagnant pool, cancerous seed cells gain a foothold and start to multiply. The gist of qigong healing is twofold—dredge the stagnation and destroy the site of cancerous growth.

A CONCISE GUIDE TO THE HEALING WALK

The following is a brief summation of the qigong healing walk practice. As with most medical therapy, the healing walk is most effective if taught by a trained expert in qigong. With qigong's growing popularity in the West and the Americas, the reader will most likely be able to find a competent qigong teacher as a guide. For the sake of readers who might not have access to such a resource, I have given an outline of the healing walk practice below. Also, I have posted several Youtube videos of my workshops on the healing walks. Although they are not instructional videos, they will give the reader a better sense of how the qigong is performed.

The video link is at http://www.qigongtherapy.com/qigong-tutorial.html

GENERAL ATTRIBUTES OF THE HEALING WALK

In essence, the healing walk is to be practiced at an unhurried pace like a languorous stroll along a riverbank or amidst a rolling wheat field in the countryside or windswept bamboo groves. As one walks, one should gaze at the far horizon. No doubt, Master Gou Lin, the creator of the Qigong walk, is encouraging patients to look far into the distant future and therefore subliminally suggesting a long life to come. So, look outward to the field afar and not at your feet!

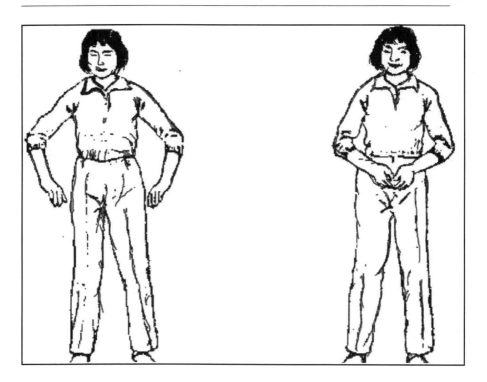

PREPARATION STANCE: THREE LINE RELAXATION

Stand naturally with feet shoulder width apart. Adjust your nose so that it lines up with your navel. Distribute your weight 50/50 between your legs. Keep your knees slightly bent as if you were standing on a seesaw.

Three Line relaxation: Imagine above the front of your head a drop of warm liquid butter dripping down the front of your body all the way to your toes. Follow the path of the butter and relax the corresponding areas of the skin, muscles and dropping your breath down as well. Now, repeat the same process but this time imagine the butter drips to the left and right side of your body and runs down your ears then to the side of the torso, and finally all the way down along your legs and to the feet. Lastly, the third line of relaxation is along the back. Visualize the warm butter slowly running down the back of your neck, oozing down along your spine and finally spreading to the left and right hamstring of your legs and pools at your heels. I find this simple short relaxation process quite beneficial in stabilizing my mind and preparing for the healing walk qigong.

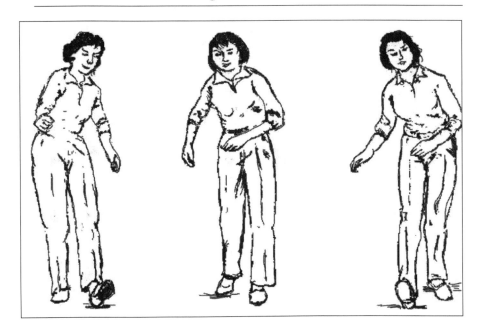

HEALING WALK QIGONG

Start by stepping with your right foot forward. Inhale, and inhale again, taking two short inhalations consecutively. Now, slowly shift weight to the right foot and gingerly roll your left foot off the floor and then take a step with your left foot forward with the left heel resting lightly on the floor, at the same time exhale once.

Now gently shift your weight to the left foot and gingerly roll your right foot-heel first, then ball and finally toe in order to step forward. As the right heel steps forward and gently touches the ground, inhale and inhale twice.

Repeat this pattern of stepping forward with the right foot with two consecutive inhalations, and then shift your weight forward and step with the left foot and exhale. After a while, you will establish an almost swimming stroke—a cycle of breath combined with the step.

Right step, inhale, inhale.

Shift weight forward to the right foot.

Left step and exhale.

Shift weight forward to the left foot.

Right step, inhale, inhale.

Shift weight forward to the right foot.

Left step and exhale.

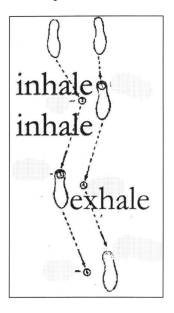

Walk in this pattern for approximately twenty minutes. take a break and rest for 10 minutes then change sides by step- ping first with your left foot.

COMPLETION AND DETOXIFICATION PROCESS

At the end of this whole segment, do the following completion movement:

First remain standing for a few moments with your eyes closed. After two to three minutes, slowly open your eyes and raise your hands over your head and then slowly squat down gently to the floor, while at the same time, let your palms press slowly along the sides of your body and imagine you are pushing out toxins from your body and organs. Simultaneously, as you squat toward the ground, make a hissing exhalation sound, which will enhance the expulsion of toxins from your body. This completion practice of the Qigong is a process of detoxification. 24 hours after chemotherapy treatment, copious amounts of saline solution were injected into my body via IV tube in order to flush out the strong toxic chemotherapeutic agents from the blood stream. Hence, the detoxification process of qigong mirrors the oncological protocol.

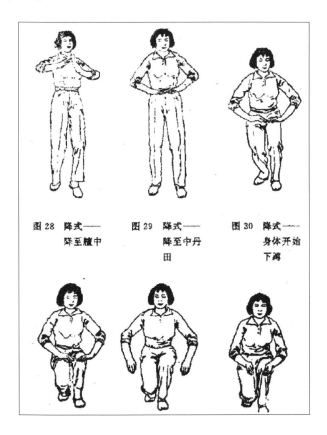

图 28　降式------
　　降至膻中

图 29　降式------
　　降至中丹
　　田

图 30　降式------
　　身体开始
　　下蹲

THE HEALING WALK QIGONG POINTERS

Turn the upper torso toward the front foot and gaze out toward the horizon and not at your foot. The Qi will follow your gaze and you don't want the Qi to go downward. A loving gaze with a soft focus allows and enhances the spread and free flow of Qi within the meridians (channels).

The kernel of the qigong walk is two inhalations and one exhalation.

In addition, swing your torso toward your leading leg, i.e. as you step with your right foot, turn your body toward the right and vice versa on the left side. Sometimes to help my beginning students, I gave them the image of a child turning her body from side to side and saying, "I don't care. I don't care." This side-to-side gyration is particularly crucial to stimulate the kidneys as well as physically squeezing out the toxic pathogens from the liver.

As for the palms' position, they should face each other like holding an invisible string between them, or imagine you are softly hugging your body. As master Gou Lin commented that this position of the palms was used to project healing Qi to our body. In TCM, the center of the palm is a powerful area called *Luo Gong,* the Chamber of Commerce, which suggests this region can project a strong life-force to others as well as to oneself. It is no wonder, that most energy healers lay their palms on their patients. By having the palms facing our body, in essence, we are projecting healing force into ourselves, to obliterate the carcinomas and to open the obstructions in our energy networks and channels.

Once in China, I observed my qigong master practicing this walk along the shore of the Pearl River; he almost looked as if he was playing and stirring a pool of water. No wonder some of my students equate the walk with swimming on land. Don't be too discouraged if you do not get it right away. No one is watching and since you are doing the qigong for healing—even done badly there will be positive affects from just the walking itself. I recall signs in the corridors of the Oncology Ward that said: Walk to health.

During one of my retreats in the South of France with my Buddhist master Thích Nhat Hanh, at the age of eighty, still lead a slow motion mindfulness walking meditation with the whole assembly of monks, nuns and lay persons. With a thousand people walking in deep awareness and total silence, I found this to be one of the most healing and moving experiences of a life time. So, don't fret excessively about whether you are doing the qigong walk correctly. Just walking slowly with deep mindfulness of your breath will surely give you great benefit. I can personally vouch for that.

If all this becomes too overwhelming, the Internet is replete with videos of cancer patients practicing their qigong walk. Simply Google the words "Gou Lin cancer walk," and you will see over 1,000 links to videos in your search results.

http://www.qigongtherapy.com/qigong-tutorial.html

FREQUENTLY ASKED QUESTIONS:

Should I breathe through the nose or mouth?

In principle, one should inhale through the nose and exhale through the mouth. However, in some cases, if your sinuses are blocked, then breathe through your mouth.

How long should I practice the walk?

Master Gou Lin has worked out a precise formula for cancer patients: walk for twenty minutes, rest for ten minutes and resume another walk for twenty minutes. On the second cycle of the walk, one should switch the lead foot, i.e. if you started with the right, change the step to begin with the left foot first.

How many times a day should I practice?

If possible, three times a day, morning, afternoon and night.

Should I eat before the qigong walk?

Yes, you should however eat a light meal. As in the previous chapter, 70% nourishment is recommended in TCM healing. Eat frequent small meals and avoid eating one or two heavy meals.

Is there any particular dietary supplement I should take?

This topic strays beyond my expertise as a qigong teacher. Notwithstanding, I can share with you my own personal dietary practice informed by my integrative oncologist, Dr. G. Cut out all refined sugar and reduce carbohydrate intake. Eat plenty of steamed vegetables especially the ones high in nutritious components such as broccoli or cauliflower. I drink a mixture of organic green tea with pomegranate powder, what Dr. G nicknamed "the purple power." As for protein, I eat mostly fish, but once in a while bone marrow soup is a great energizer and regenerative broth.

Will you tell me your integrative oncologist's name?

Unfortunately, in order to protect his privacy, I cannot. However, I can give you a hint. He lives and works in New York City and as far as I know, he is the one and only integrative oncologist who has a clinical practice in New York City.

Where can I find a competent qigong teacher in my area?

Personally, I searched for almost a decade to find my Taoist master weeding through a field of charlatans and mediocre teachers. In most cases, word of mouth from other students is the best resource for finding a teacher. A Chinese master who lacks rudimentary English will not be a good guide for English speakers. As I am a native of China, my Chinese master was a wonderful and generous teacher; however, for his western students he lacked the ability to communicate the depth and profundity of the qigong practice. Hence, many of his western students only received a superficial understanding of qigong.

Avoid the zealots who extol exaggerated methods such as excessive fasting or extreme vegetarianism as sole alternatives to cure cancer. I walked down that path with nearly fatal results. One popular qigong master with no medical training even prohibited his students from seeking chemotherapy or radiation. His layman's reason is that since cancer patients already suffer from a deficient immune system, it would be too injurious to their defenses. He also practices a form of external Qi emission that can supposedly disperse carcinomas; this is an intriguing yet clinically unproven methodology. Personally, I chose the complementary approach using chemotherapy in conjunction with holistic practices. Therefore I recommend finding a qigong master who views his or her practice as complementary to standard medical treatment. I am living proof of this approach and one of the reasons for this book is to share my experience with others. Even my regular oncologist Dr. M proclaimed, "In spite of all the toxic chemicals we threw at you, you managed to sail through the treatment without any adverse side effects." However, you don't have to limit yourself to only one modality.

Can I come and study with you?

I would, with all my heart, love to say "yes". However, I live and work in a modest private studio in New York City, and it would be logistically impossible to accept the massive demand of cancer patients. Yet another reason for this book is to share this practice with a wider audience. I intend to hold public seminars and workshops on qigong healing, so please consult my website (www.qigongtherapy.com) for upcoming events.

Any final words to help me in the fight against my particular cancer?

Know that you have a healing power within you and all the doctors, healing herbs and treatments are but complementary to your own spontaneous healing force. Moreover, healing does not necessarily mean only curing the disease, rather healing takes place when you are at peace with the outcome of illness and joyful knowing that you have done all that you can to fight the disease. Thus failure is not an option and success possible in every step along the way. Don't ever give up hope. In the words of the immortal Ralph Waldo Emerson, "Life must be lived on a higher plain, to which we are always invited to ascend; there, the whole aspect of things changes."

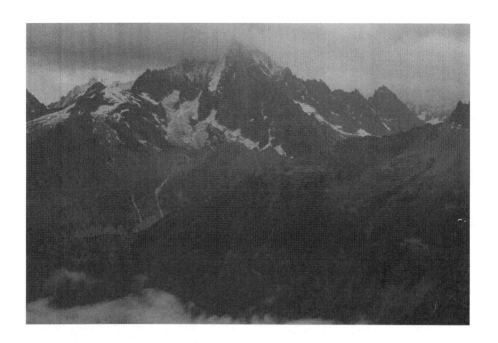

CHAPTER TEN: THE CURE

"You sailed through chemotherapy," Dr. M commented as he examined me, probing deep inside the axillary lymph nodes under my armpits. "I could tell my patients to do exercises, but I can't guide them towards the type of exercise that might be most appropriate for their particular kind of cancer." He sighed under his breath. I witnessed a little flicker of his eyes; perhaps a Nordic understated mannerism, like a Butoh dancer conveying a depth of emotion with only the most infinitesimal movement.

My wife Janet observed from the sidelines amazed at the exchange between us. "He is basking in your presence..." She paused slightly then continuing her thought, "It must be quite a heavy burden to work with late-stage cancer patients. You must be a breath of fresh air to him."

This was the final PET scan. With my cancer completely vanquished, I no longer needed a clinical scan, but rather just a watchful eye and a physical exam every three to four months for a period of eighteen months. I caught a glimpse of laughter appearing around the corner of Janet's lips as Dr. M relayed the news to us. After two years remaining free of any cancerous cells, this particular cancer will not return for life, therefore, my cancer is cured. The alchemy of healing cancer diverges into myriad streams, but in essence, cancer treatment can be divided into four categories: curable, incurable but treatable, untreatable and terminal, untreatable and slow growth. Within these four types, I am very fortunate to have the curable kind, Large B-cell Lymphoma.

THE WHOLE PATH LAID OUT (IN RETROSPECT)

As I recall the events of the past as reflected in the convex mirror of my memory, I ardently hope no mistakes have been made and that each step I took was full of clarity and well intended. The truth is far from this mirror of perfection. I stumbled and fumbled my way toward the discovery and treatment of my cancer. I committed the initial mistake of minimizing the symptoms of the oral tumor as a mere abscess. It was only by the careful concern of my dentist in trying to excise the abscess (which did not behave like one) was I sent to an oral surgeon for a biopsy.

At the crux of it all, I realized that cancer exists outside the realm of common diseases. I did not feel sick or weakened by the growth of the cancerous tumor, but it was only insofar as the tumor distorted my face into what my wife so bluntly described as "simian" that I began to see the problem with greater clarity. As one cancer researcher put it, "Cancer is composed entirely of real estate issues." One doesn't die of cancer, but the disease literally pushes one out of one's own body. Our organs are squeezed by the fecund growth of the carcinoma and therefore no longer function properly. Hence, cancer could be viewed as rapidly reproducing locusts that eat and destroy everything in sight.

Of course, in hindsight, being trained as a Chinese doctor, I should have been able to recognize the symptoms much earlier. Therefore, in my case this axiom is more than appropriate: the patient who treats himself has an imbecile for a doctor. Utterly true!

Instead, in self-delusion, I fumbled down alternative routes to heal my cancer with more natural means. As one of my colleagues in holistic medicine succinctly put it, "If we who have practiced and taught holistic, alternative medicine for a lifetime jumped ship at the first sign of cancer, that would not do." Henceforth, I charged headlong into the gale armed with nothing more than my qigong and TCM training. I was swept in the passing darkness of fear and denial. My poor wife loyally followed and supported my path whereas my daughters, observing from the clarity of the sidelines, saw my fear and denial vividly. One of the initial holistic healers I consulted equated cancer with nothing more than a "bicycle accident" and that one shouldn't be "obsessed with the carcinomas". But the tumors started to swell and gain in size almost daily.

Drawing from my training, I know that cancer is due to a weakened body and polluted environment. My life was filled with the stresses of a successful healing practice and I had just returned to a master's program in acupuncture full-time. My diet was filled with the usual sugar saturated items of a fast-food culture such as donuts, cookies and ice cream. Unbeknownst to me, at that point, the cancerous cells were already placing a demand on my body to consume copious amounts of sugar to fuel their unceasing, rapid cellular growth.

My first act was to cleanse my body with a twenty-one day fast eating only one bowl of bone marrow soup daily. Furthermore, I removed all sugar, including orange juice from my diet, and I have been able to maintain this sugar-free diet to date. This cleansing was instrumental in strengthening my body and preparing it for the chemotherapy to come. I feel that it contributed to my total lack of nausea and helped with the side effects from the treatment. A note of caution to the readers: this is an acute drastic cleansing diet and can be, to a certain extent, very dangerous due to the concentrated release of accrued toxins from the fat cells of your own body. In a recent example, a dozen seals were found dead of poisoning on the California coast. Forensic examination revealed that due to an extended period of food deprivation due to storms, their fatty tissues were metabolized rapidly releasing their previously accumulated toxins. As a consequence, they were poisoned by their own body's stored toxic waste. Thus readers must have a competent nutritionist to guide them towards the means to protect themselves against this common toxic release syndrome.

In retrospect, my critical assessment of myself during this time was that I was stubborn in my strict adherence to alternative medicine and my dogged belief that it alone would cure me. I had mistaken faith in oneself for the science of healing. Only by the grace of my daughters' intervention was I able to switch over to the complementary modality of cancer treatment. I recollect distinctly a crisp, chilly fall afternoon, waiting in line with my eldest daughter for the bus as she was then working in Boston. She had celebrated her twenty-second birthday and when I asked her what birthday gift I could give her, she replied, "See an oncologist." This was her one request and I promised.

Halfheartedly, I scheduled an appointment with Dr. G more to satisfy my daughters' demands than anything else. My youngest threatened never to return home from college, and my middle daughter kept encouraging me to confront and face my fear. My decision to see an integrative oncologist was intended, more than anything else, to empower and heal my daughters. Deep in my heart I knew how much my sickness had impacted my family; it was like a bullet hitting and fracturing a panel of glass. I didn't want my daughters to undergo the descent into utter helplessness. So almost three months from the date of the discovery of cancer, I met Dr. G and crossed into a complementary medicine in order to treat my cancer. Finally, I started chemotherapy the second week of October 2010. As they say, the rest is history.

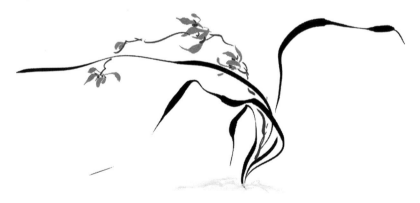

THE AWAKENED STATE OF BEING

"So irresistible is the transformative power of enlightenment that your life seems to shift into a new dimension, open to new and unsuspected possibilities."

—Eugene Herrigel, The Method of Zen, 1960,

Being a Buddhist, every aspect of life, especially the fundamental sufferings of birth, sickness, old age and death, serve as opportunities for awakening. All along, from the very moment my cancer was first discovered, to the treatment and finally the curing of the disease, I seized each stage as an unfolding of a process to open and reveal my true self-nature—the Buddha within. This sentiment helped me to transcend the confines of my own individual drama and open to a larger spiritual realm, ultimately propelling me to face my personal demons. I feel that this singular factor is an important contribution to my healing, and gives me the possibility to move beyond personal tragedy to universality—allowing a wider perspective and the inclusion of humanity. By letting go of my attachment to a small self, I gain the whole world. The essence of our awakened nature is a boundless being with an intrinsic quality of unbearable lightness. In the metaphorical language of Indian mythology, from the body of a sleeping Krishna grows a singular lotus which blossoms into the universe; this awakened Buddha nature is the Godhead. This lightness of being is enlightenment in every moment, an instantaneous awakening beyond any notion of time and space. For enlightenment is not a fixed state but rather the essence of our true-self, an evanescence of the spirit—an infinite ever-widening sense of the unfathomable consciousness. This field of energy manifests in matters of the heart, the light and the darkness of our human nature. Our ordinary consciousness is part of this infinite awakened nature, yet it is enshrouded or hidden by the ego's tendency to fragment, and thus creating the illusion of a separate self-existence. The analogy of a white light that unifies all colors into a single luminosity is our radiant awakened nature. As this light of awareness descends into the daily struggles of survival and search for pleasure it refracts into myriad parts creating a multifaceted mirage called the "ego" with its agitating, grasping, pretense and beliefs.

The color of gold is also a manifestation of this white light. In the Garland School of Buddhist practice, the golden lion is formed from the substance of gold yet the object, the lion does not exist apart from its substance. The gold serves as its true nature; imagine melting the golden lion, the gold still exist as substance. Thus, the substance of gold can take many shapes and forms, producing the arising of various images whether it be a Buddha, lions, or angels without separate existence. The arising and melting of these golden creatures are analogous to the billions of births and deaths of human beings on this earth, yet our true essence or being; the immortal gold nature remains utterly unchanged and is beyond life, death, sickness and old age. Hence, the process of enlightenment is to plunge and awaken this nature of being. Unfortunately, the human language especially the Indo-European tongue has already evolved with the egotistic, possessive pronouns of mine, yours, his, hers, theirs and ours. In 'Being,' there is no such place for a possessive pronoun. To conceive of the awakened nature belonging to a fragmentary self is completely nonsensical and ultimately a form of insanity. Therefore, the phrase, 'I am enlightened' is an oxymoron for in the enlightening state of being all identification and separation dissolves into the vast cosmic ocean of consciousness. There is only awakened nature without coloration or image, there is only enlightening without the 'I am.'

Cultivation in inner alchemy involves seeing our subtle nature of breath and sexuality. Thus, in inner alchemy, the feminine is not outside of man but exists in the very in-breath of SA. The mantra, SA, represents the feminine principle of spirit and is infused into the sexual center of the abdominal region. During exhalation, the mantra Ham is released in orgasmic union with the Void, the supreme emptiness of Wuji. Hence, a single breath composed of inhalation and exhalation, is transformed into a cosmic dance of unification with the Divine, the creative principle of Tao. However, this sublime dance eludes the ordinary person in his/her attachment to the body, or thought patterns composed of purely biological processes. The alchemy of healing does not manifest if the subtle bodies, the river of consciousness and life forces become stagnant.

For me, I came upon such realization after a sleepless night at the isolation unit of the ER when every part of me was utterly exhausted and all the operators of my cunning mind ceased, and within this still-point of complete silence, I gazed back at my own original unborn face. Instantaneously, I was plunged into a boundless, non-conceptual consciousness and the mind stopped; time stood still, space expanded then vanished. All that was left is pure un-fabricated pristine awareness without self, other or anything else. In that brief moment perhaps lasting no longer than a few minutes, my life had irrevocably shifted from insanity to sanity, from the delusion of ego-hood to boundless being. And I wept and then laughed: So that's it. *Tat Tvam Asi.* Suchness. Enlightenment. Awake!

From that moment on, life genuinely has taken on a wholly other dimension as if stepping out of a black-and-white film into the techno-color radiance of vivid senses. It is difficult to describe but the sensation is of having managed somehow to break through the air-bubble of self-protection into wide-open space. Fear, passions and the pursuit of things still inhabit me, yet they have lost their barb and sharp edges. Things that used to deeply trouble me no longer tug at me in the same way. My skin feels fresh with a tender tingling sensation as I reach out with fingers trembling in front touching the uncertainty of the unknown.

From this vantage point on, my meditation takes on a wholly different timbre, no longer am I obsessed with the search for enlightenment, the awakening to the Self; rather, as I sit on the cushion, it is just plain abiding in my Self-nature; within this formless boundless awareness, all struggles to become cease.

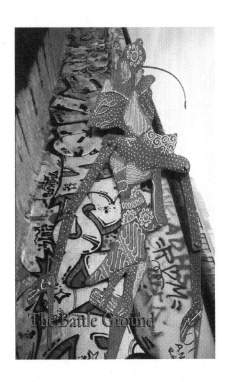

The Battle Ground

Chapter Eleven:
Post Traumatic Stress

Post Traumatic Stress

Every year at the time of my annual check-up with my oncologist, my body and mind go through a reflexive sense of dread. Past memories of sleeplessly strolling along the hospital corridor like a solitary swimmer swimming lap after lap in a narrow pool. The sound of beeping, interspersed with the hidden groans and moans from shuttered rooms all percolate up in a pungent acrid haze like the steamy spirit rising up from a hot asphalt road in the Arizona desert.

Post-Traumatic Stress Syndrome (PTSS) is a gnawing recurrence of fear and anxiety. I still get PTSS around the time of my periodic PET scan. One of my patients, a Vietnam War veteran who had his legs blown off by a land-mine would collapse at the sound of a car backfiring, similarly my internal body's remembrance of the different sensations I had while infected with cancer will trigger panic. This recurrence is a natural part of the healing process and something to be witnessed. The knowledge of this relieves me of the anxiety.

HOW TO DEAL WITH PTSS?

In a recent trip to Berlin, I visited the Jewish Museum; it is one of the largest Jewish Museums in Europe. In three buildings, two of which are new additions specifically built for the museum by architect Daniel Libeskind, two millennia of German-Jewish history are on display in the permanent exhibition as well as in various changing exhibitions. Just outside of the building is the remnant of the original Berlin Wall. In a single location, we have both memories of two epic tragedies: the holocaust and the artificial separation of a community drawn by political lines. So what do these two memorials stand for? The answer that came to me is that they are healing centers for a communities' collective PTSS as well as reminders of the tragic stupidity of humanity. Watching the long lines of young and old shuffle along the wall, walking down the same cobble stone path as their ancestors, I could almost see the invisible healing forces being soaked into their bodies from the ground. Perhaps some must be seek forgiveness; others search for a way to reconcile the abrupt rift of a family suddenly torn apart. From the Taoist shamanic healing perspective, places of trauma also possess healing power. A survivor of Auschwitz once told me that for decades she resisted going back to the death camp. She was haunted by vivid recurring nightmares and a deep sense of survivor's guilt (why had she survived and not her family?). Her life was racked with daily torment and clinical depression. Only at the urging of her Rabbi did she finally agree to return to the death camp. The first time she stepped foot on the camp grounds her whole body started to shiver and tremble uncontrollably and then she fainted. That night she sobbed; she felt forgiveness from her mother who had died from one of those 'showers'. In her dream, she felt her mother whispering in her ear and stroking her hair the way she used to when she was a little girl. And for the first time in her life, she slept without nightmares.

As part of my Taoist healing practice, I have come to treat a wide range of clients who have suffered from PTSS. From the perspective that the place of trauma is also the location for healing, I recommend many of my clients who suffer from PTSS to visit the site of the tragedy. In most cases, they come to profound revelations regarding the incident that they had tried to suppress from their minds. These insights give meaning to their inner fear and guilt, and through our work together we slowly unwind the psychic entanglement that caused their heart and mind to twist into a knot. For readers, I would like to impose a word of caution: Do not attempt to try this on your own. It is dangerous to return to the site of ground zero without a competent healer to empower you, for surely this place will trigger extremely strong emotional responses or even physical symptoms.

For myself, I have devised a little prayer that I often repeat in times of stress and PTSS.

With an overwhelming sense of gratitude and celebration of life, I embrace each moment. I experience the full glory of pain, anguish and ecstasy—the full palate of colors composing the rainbow of consciousness. Thus, in feeling the pain of loss, the fear of one's mortality, I enjoy each part of the landscape of life.

RECOVERY FROM PTSS

My late master once told me that as a healer I would encounter patients who would exhibit the very ailments that I might have and healing them would allow my own healing as well. The old saying 'healer heal thyself' is put into a whole other perspective. Thus, as I began to heal my own PTSS, many clients who exhibited Post-Traumatic symptoms appeared at my doorstep.

I am very fortunate indeed to have had the opportunity to heal myself. In one recent case, one of three American hikers imprisoned in Iran on suspicion of espionage came to me for treatment. In the book, *A Sliver of Light: Three Americans imprisoned in Iran,* Joshua relates his story of being imprisoned and the loss that ensued as his body no longer seemed to belong to him but rather to the prison guards. Having all his clothes stripped away and replaced with prison garb and being blind folded the guards started to spin him in circles. Then he was suddenly shoved into a bare 8 by 12 foot cell. As I see it, this was way the Iranian guards' stripped away all of Joshua's sense of self and self control. Joshua felt that his body was theirs. He had inexplicably lost himself.

But the road back from an Iranian jail cell—where he spent more than two years—to a life in the United States has been filled with thorns and obstacles. The central issue for Joshua was not only the loss of freedom but also the loss of self. In order to heal from his ordeal he would need to recover his own sense of self and self-control. I feel an incredible privilege to be able to accompany Joshua along this long road toward healing. One vignette that I found especially valuable for my PTSS clients is to see the rose amidst the thorns. In our work together, Joshua came to see that his suffering serves as a reminder of the preciousness of freedom and that in a small way, he and his fellow hikers contributed to the negotiations between Iran, the United States and five other countries regarding the future of the Iranian nuclear program. As a result, Tehran would dismantle parts of its nuclear infrastructure in exchange for the lifting of sanctions, according to a statement released in Vienna by all seven nations. And that undeniably, would be quite a rose.

Finally being freed from the tiny Iranian prison cell, Joshua found the world almost frighteningly immense and unconsciously he persisted to return to confined spaces. The dark shadows of the Iranian prison guards were ghoulish apparitions that upon his return shape-shifted into the officials at the motor vehicle department, the landlord's office or the bank, and everywhere Joshua heard the same refrains that were repeated by the Iranian guards: "I don't know. You'll have to talk to my boss. He is not in right now."

It enraged him that physically free he was still caught in a mental prison cell.

Then he was reunited with his childhood sweetheart, Jenny. Their relationships was a breath of fresh air completely different from the time of his imprisonment with his cell mate, the prison guards or the interrogators. He didn't have to use the drastic measures of a hunger strike or bang on the cell door to be heard, and this new way of love opened a whole other dimension of delight as well as complications.

Writing his recollection for his book, *A Sliver of Light,* Joshua came to the passage about how Shane and their bickering over the petty details of their tiny cell, and then for no particular rhyme or reason he would get angry with Jenny for how she looked, for the way she sighed and for leaving the bathroom light on. He didn't stop until she yelled, "I'm not Shane!" Suddenly, he realized that he had a PTSS episode and decided to seek therapy. Through working together Joshua and I were able to untangle some of the patterns and release traumatic residual shadows that lingered and at times reemerged.

"...After years of feeling utterly unsettled, I sensed I was now exactly where I should be. Finding love helped me find my way amid the tangles of history, and it helped Jenny and me secure a place in the world where, like the aptly titled play from our childhood, we were free to be a family..." Reaching Out Between the Bars by Joshua Fattal, NOV. 20, 2014, Nytimes article

The potential for recovery is always present. Against all odds and prospects, our lives take an unforeseen turn and suddenly the grace of release is received and we are once again whole, totally healed from within. Only then, will the phantoms of past trauma utterly evaporate like the morning mist on an Adirondack lake and perhaps this is why we meditate. Meditation is not intended to actively pursue healing from PTSS, but it cultivates a willing and receptive openness that allows the possibility of grace to enter. This kind of healing does not arise from any internal or external forces. This seemingly passive approach is not for the impatient person and therefore most inevitably would choose a more direct frontal solution to resolve the residual traumatic stress. Still, I cherish the sliver of solitude, a meditation; I hope, more than anything, this will bring the joy of life and the release we so ardently search for.

Here, then, is the way of alchemical meditation which will allow the blossoming of equanimity. It is a crucial aspect of healing; in a state of stillness and tranquility one absorbs energy from the universal, dark matter. In fact the ancient Taoists discovered that this energy is plentiful in the cosmos and ripe for the taking. However, if your mind is turbulent like a shaking teacup as tea is being poured into it, you will in likelihood receive a meager cup of tea indeed. The abundance of energy surrounding us is rather astonishing. For the Taoists, meditation is not a process simply to become relaxed, or as in the Buddhist context, a way towards enlightenment. Rather, alchemical meditation is a direct way to absorb the healing Qi that surrounds us. Closely aligned with Taoist healing principles is ancient Ayurvedic medicine and it has four fundamental elements: ether, water, fire and earth. Hence, I see a correlation with Taoist concept of qi as the etheric energy that arises out of nothing. During my overly zealous apprenticeship, my teacher would gently admonish me, "Sitting in a state of turmoil and exertion is a waste of time. It is as if you are shaking a screaming child to calm her down. Only when you drop both your mind and body, letting them fall like autumn leaves, will the sublime iridescent Qi enter and dispel the dark pathogens and negative emotions which lurk in your body." Finally in the light of meditation the shadowy assassin, PTSS, has met its match.

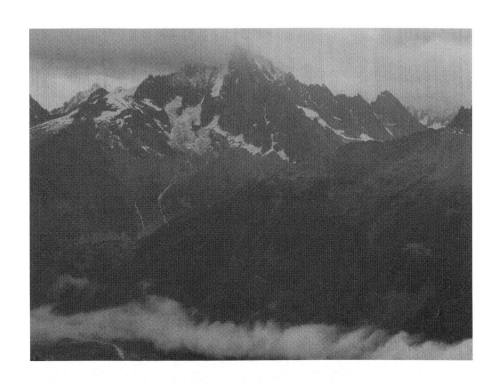

Chapter Twelve:
The Last Frontier

The Future of Cancer Treatment, Recovery & Prevention

The story of cancer begins at the dawn of humanity and takes a headlong plunge like Alice in Wonderland wandering a circuitous path. Each passing generation of surgeons, oncologists, scientists and patients clamor for the cancer cure. Similar to the strangeness of Wonderland, the story of cancer is filled with bizarre desperation as in the cases of the mad Egyptian queen ordering her slave to cut off her cancerous breasts, or the quixotic Dr. Halsted with his radical surgery excising all traces of cancerous tissues to the point of irrevocably maiming a patient's body. As we look back, we remain aghast at the cruelty of these draconian measures that defy common sense or healing or the possibility of being whole. They are the products of false premises and heuristic judgment by overenthusiastic surgeons and scientists in their excessive compassion to win the war against cancer; when, in truth, the identity of the enemy has not yet been clearly seen. In this case, the old adage, "Don't shoot before you see the whites of your enemy's eyes," has not been heeded. Clinicians are far too quick to order any sort of last resort treatment for a dying patient. Their grief-stricken families cling to experimental trials as their last straw of hope.

To envision the future of cancer treatment, recovery and prevention is to re-imagine the possibility of seeing the whites of our foe's fiery eyes. Cancer is a genetic disease of mutation. The tools of surgery, radiation and chemotherapy are too blunt to wield the necessary mortal blows at the microscopic level that genes require. Therefore, the future of cancer treatment lies in gene repair protocols and identifying the unique DNA sequence of each cancer. Oncologist must learn to attack the very genetic code of cancer cells directly. Out of this approach, innovative therapies have emerged, such as the use of antibodies and a genetically engineered HIV retrovirus to infiltrate the cancerous DNA codes resulting in some remarkable success. These are some of the first nonlethal precision treatments that do not wipe out whole classes of cells as in the case of chemotherapy. Targeted gene therapy is yielding many low-hanging fruit in the use of anti-clone bodies such as Retuxan or other treatments that zoom in on cancer cells and tag them for the immune cells to eradicate later. As genetic research and mapping become more efficient and available, future patients will most likely have the genetic code of their individual cancer cells all mapped out and oncologists will then be able to predict and identify the behaviors and reactions of the cancer cells to chemo treatments.

Additionally, a holistic approach to cancer treatment will be incorporated in the overall plan of action to heal cancer. Initial research on qigong and Taiji from China and the National Institute of Health (NIH) has indicated their effectiveness in helping to heal cancer as well as depression. In the process of treating the body, we should not neglect the mind and spirit of the cancer patient. A holistic approach from alternative medicine fields should be folded into the overall treatment plan. And in the following section, I will present my own personal self-experimentation on using this Complementary Therapeutic approach. Lucky for me, the outcome was wildly successful.

Toward a Complementary Therapeutic Approach

Having been my own Guinea pig, I will delineate what I have done in complement with standard medical cancer treatment for my lymphoma.

Foremost in my healing strategy was the positive support and faith of my wife and daughters. Upon hearing that I had cancer, my eldest daughter predicted that I would write a bestseller, a memoir of my experience in recovering from cancer. I then promised that I would share 10% of the royalties from the book with her. This positive outlook was crucial during my treatment, uplifting me during the exceedingly difficult and dangerous procedures. Her prediction empowered me to take center stage in my battle against this disease.

After the initial diagnoses I did not rush for treatment. I wanted to have a second opinion from an integrative oncologist who was more allied with my holistic medical background and sensibility. During this twilight period, I started a fast and cleansing diet, detoxifying for twenty-one days. In Taoist healing this is called Bigu, which literally means shutting out any ingestion of grain and food. I modified the routine by having a bowl of bone marrow soup seasoned with ample amounts of seaweed, ginger and garlic every morning. This protocol enhanced the detoxification along with replenishing nutritious elements within the body. At the hospital before any chemo treatment was administered, the initial marker of my cancer was taken. During this first round of tests, my cancer index was 7 to 8. In comparison, my roommate who had the same type of Lymphoma, his index was in the 60's. One of the interns at the hospital was impressed that I had such a low cancer count. Secretly, I felt that my low index might be due to the initial Bigu fast/cleansing diet. Certainly, by having cleansed my body of the most toxic stagnation, my reaction to the chemo treatment was, as Dr. M put it, "Not Interesting!" Having your oncologist proclaimed that your blood work in response to the chemo treatment was utterly uninteresting is a good thing. Therefore, I was able to sail through the twelve cycles of highly toxic chemo treatment without even the slightest nausea, hiccup or organ damage.

BONE MARROW SOUP RECIPE

2 lb. of organic and grass fed beef soup bones

3 cloves of garlic

3 slices of ginger

1 onion (or soaked Kombu seaweed)

2 table spoon of Olive oil

1 large pot of water - 8 cups

Cooking:

Heat the olive oil in a large pot. Place the garlic, ginger and chopped onion or (soaked overnight Kombu) in the pot. Let it simmer for 30 seconds. Place the beef bones in the pot and brown them-this will seal in the juice. Pour water into the pot and bring to a boil. Lower the flame and cover the pot, let it simmer for 4 hours.(Add water if too much liquid has been evaporated.) Ready to be served. Let it cool down to room temperature. Any leftover can be stored in a glass jar in the refrigerator for the next several days.

ACUPUNCTURE

Acupuncture is an ancient Chinese therapeutic technique for relieving pain, curing disease, and improving general health. We now know that it was devised before 2500 BC in China as remnants of stone acupuncture needles have been discovered in Neolithic Caves. By the late 20th century, acupuncture became widely accepted in many countries of the global community. The United States is one of the first countries to establish a state license for acupuncturist as independent medical therapists in treating diseases without medical drugs. Acupuncture consists of the insertion of one or several small metal needles into the skin and underlying tissues at defined points on the body.

Acupuncture grew out of Taoist philosophy's complementary cosmic forces of the yin and the yang. The yin, the feminine principle, is receptive and dark; it corresponds to the Earth's quality of gentleness and carries the burden of nourishing all life. The yang, the masculine principle, is strong and light and is denoted by the heaven's everlasting dynamic motion. The forces of yin and yang interact in the human body as they do throughout the natural universe as a whole. Within our body, blood is regarded as yin and cooling, while breath/Qi is considered to be yang and warming. Disease or physical disharmony is caused by an imbalance or undue preponderance of these two forces in the body, and the goal of Chinese medicine is to bring the yin and the yang back into harmony and thus re-establish the individual's health.

For me, personally, I found that acupuncture reduced my nausea to zero. It was quite a sight, to see me sticking my body full of needles while getting chemo treatments at the hospital. It was to a certain extent wonderful to have acupuncture on demand. One time, my roommate asked me whether I could treat him, but I had to decline, for at that point; I was a little busy healing myself.

QIGONG

Qigong walks became for me the life-line, the central exercise at the hospital and at home. The particular qigong walk is remarkably beneficial in expelling chemo's toxic substances from the body. Unbeknownst to many cancer patients, twenty-four hours after the chemo is injected into the body; the toxins have done their job of killing the cancerous cells and therefore, after this period, they should be expunged as quickly as possible. One should drink ample fluids as well as exercise to speed up the process. I was able within a twenty-four-hour period to expel 99.9% of the chemo and in another twenty-four hours 99.99% of the chemo was expunged.

MEDITATION

Meditation is akin to sunlight, a daily dose of meditation will spread a sheen of peace and joy in all activities including the monotonous details required in cancer treatment. My life was chopped up into small slices of twenty-one days and taking the time to meditate allowed me to transcend (at least during those meditative moments) the concerns of sickness and despair. My meditation was composed of silent seated meditation as well as watching a film on my IPad about the life of the Buddha. In some ways, seeing the Buddha walk along the path of liberation from the suffering of birth, old age, sickness and death, comforted me as I dealt with my own sickness and possible imminent death.

NUTRITION

Having a nutritious diet is critical in fighting cancer. I took a unique formula of vitamins, fruit powders and vegetables as prescribed by my integrative Oncologist, Dr. G. Here is an absolutely critical point: one must have a trained professional prescribe such dietary supplements. Dr. G had decades of training in this field of integrative medicine. One of his patients with terminal pancreatic cancer was able to extend her life way beyond the prognosis of her regular oncologist who had given her six months at the utmost to live. Five years later, I met her at Dr. G's office for my annual checkup.

Last, but not least, maintain an overall positive attitude that everything you have done will contribute to your healing; this mind-set will ignite your spontaneous healing power. Then everything serves you in your healing journey. From my personal experience working with cancer patients, most people with cancer and their oncologists are leery of unreachable expectations so as not to be disappointed. With such a mind-set, they are unconsciously shifting their mental attitude towards a pessimistic one and thereby putting themselves at a disadvantage. I suggest that you not bear such 'realistic' burdens but let your oncologist shoulder this responsibility. Thus, as a patient, your sole task is to live as fully and as carefree as possible; you just live your life completely with a sense of grace—that every moment is a gift from heaven. Let the doctors worry about you.

An extraordinary paradigm of such positive and wild courage is Kris Carr's film, *Crazy Sexy Cancer*, which documented her journey after being diagnosed with untreatable, stage 4 cancer. She began a health revolution by refusing to sink to the pessimism and overly 'realistic' attitude of some of her oncologists. The ones who told her to have a double organ transplant she fired. Eight years later, Kris is still alive and married which explains why you shouldn't be afraid to dream big. Bravo to Ms. Carr for her outrageous courage and positive attitude. For she is not only able to maintain a healthy life but has inspired a multitude of cancer patients to emerge from the shadow of dark depression and pessimism to the sunny side of laughter, joy and aliveness.

HOW DOES IT FEEL TO HAVE YOUR CANCER CURED?

I am often asked, "How does it feel to have your cancer cured?" And in response I am taken, once again, by a wave of sensation that rises in my belly and washes over my vision with a kind of burning. I want to answer with something more, something that goes beyond the common simple emotions, expressed by the refrain "I am so happy and lucky." What I want to say has to do with all the people who have died—the ones who did not make it or the little girl who gave me a thumbs up in chemo. However, I also feel my own incredible good fortune at having overcome the close call of devastating loss. So, my response is not only connected with the celebration of life—the joy of living, but is also inevitably related to the penetrating constant shadow of unavoidable death. When the light burns bright so does the shadow grow.

I would say that this feeling is akin to an experience I had two summers ago when my wife and I scaled a mountain in the French Alps. It was an ascent filled with narrow ledges where one must use the iron chain-link embedded in the rock face to pull oneself up the cliff, or traverse a mountain stream that falls precipitously down to a misty dark abyss. "Don't look down" was no comfort as one skipped over small gaps between river stones. And then near the peak, the rolls of thunder moved closer and heavy droplets of rain started to pelt down. My thigh muscles, the quadriceps, had given up a few miles back and only through pure mental force could I will them to move. With the high altitude, my lungs started to hurt and my heart raced. Being trained in physical medicine, I knew full well all the symptoms of hypothermia. My body began to shiver uncontrollably and quite paradoxically; I felt a giddy sense of humor about the whole thing. It was supposedly just a quaint little hike along a mountain trail. Somehow, an image arose from Hemingway's *The Snows of Kilimanjaro*, when close to the western summit they came across, a dried, frozen carcass of a leopard. As I laughed out loud, Janet turned around in deep concern. One step at a time, urged my mountain guide gently. I could no longer feel any sensation in my toes and had to use my eyes to watch where I placed my feet; I stepped gingerly like a ballerina pointing her toe shoes. Internally, I felt as if the biological gauge of my reserves had its needle rapidly lowering into the red zone and started to blink: empty! empty! Then, suddenly, the mountain refuge appeared just around the bend in the trail, behind this rustic lodge were frosty glacial peaks stood like granite sentinels with the last salmon-pink sunset behind them. I collapsed on the trail and literally crawled my final hundred feet up to the refuge. Inside the warm dry chalet, the guardians were serving hot butternut squash soup and homemade bread. Right there and then, I knew, as I realize now, this is how I must reply to the question "how do you feel now that your cancer is cured?"

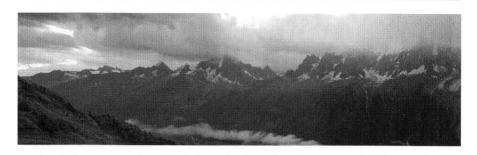

THE MOUNTAIN REFUGE

Almost at the point of collapse, blinding exhaustion

this appears
and one is delirious giddy
exhilarated

dancing in the throne of Gods

My heart opens
honey amber sap flows out
and soaks the silver creeks
glistening boulders

Tiny lavender trumpet-flowers
quiver ever so slightly
as I stumble
stagger
crawl my way up the Mountain Refuge

—at the Summit near Mount Blanc

ACKNOWLEDGEMENTS

Foremost, I would like to express my gratitude to my wife and fellow 'hitchhiker', Janet, who has been a constant companion in my life and by my side during my hospital stays. Some days, she would visit me twice and bring the life-saving chicken broth. I am also deeply grateful to my daughters who banded together in a united front to persuade me toward the complementary path of both chemotherapy as well as holistic healing. I wish to thank my student and editor, Alicia Fox, who not only stayed with me during my time of tribulation and darkness, but also worked faithful to put my words into a clear voice.

In having cured my cancer, I owe my life literally to my two outstanding oncologists, Dr. Peter Martin and Dr. Mitchell Gaynor who guided me and helped me to cross over. Their dedication as physicians and their compassionate humanity is both humbling and inspiring. During the black out of Hurricane Sandy, Dr. Martin rode his bicycle all the way from lower Manhattan through the black-out streets to the hospital on 68th street to see patients; one of them was me. Of course, Dr. Martin would not have considered such an act as anything special; he would probably say, "I'm just doing my job." And the staff and nurses at the Weill-Cornell Medical College Oncology Unit, showed such cheerfulness and caring in the face of cancer.

Also, I owe a depth of gratitude to my longtime student of more than two decades and colleague, Dr. Adriano Borgna, who is a physician (Italy), an acupuncturist and sublime chef. During my initial rude awakening of discovering the cancer, he showed me great kindness and encouraged a positive outlook in combating the cancer. He taught me how to cook the bone marrow soup.

In addition, I am eternally grateful for my own personal healer and longtime student, Barbara K., in giving me regular treatments in Medical Qigong which I had taught her. Under her healing and care, I could almost feel the chemotherapy toxins being leached from my body. Conceivably, this could be viewed as a karmic cycle of the student healing the teacher.

Last but not least, one other student, Aaron Sternberg, deserves my deep gratitude for his immaculate devotion and support during my stays at the hospital. Not only would he bring the healing broth of chicken soup, he sometimes even walked with me in the Healing Walk and inevitably, other cancer patients would join in. I am so blessed to have him guarding my back and supporting me in spreading the message and teaching of CHA.

BIBLIOGRAPHY

Emperor of All Maladies: A Biography of Cancer by Siddhartha Mukherjee, Published by Scribner Publication. 2010

"Forty Years' War on Cancer" series from The New York Times by Gina Kolata, Published: April 23, 2009

The Secret History of the War on Cancer by Devra Davis, Published by Basic Books, October 2007

黄帝内经, Huangdi Neijing, *The Yellow Emperor's Treatise on Internal Medicine* (475-221 BC).

Science and Civilisation in China fifth volume, Alchemy by Joseph Needham, Cambridge University Press; First Edition; Later Printing edition (August 14, 1954).

静坐修道与长生不老, *Tao of Longevity* by 南怀瑾, Nan Huai-Chin, published by Samuel Weiser Books, Boston, MA, 1994

郭林气功全集，*Complete Works of Gou Lin New Qigong Therapy*, edited by 吴承, Wu Zhen Wei, Beijing Gou Lin Qigong Institute, 1990

刘太医谈养生: Royal Physician Lu's Reflections on Nourishing Life, by 刘弘章, Lu Huang Zhiang, 刘浡, Lu Hu 著. Published by 中国友谊出版公司, China Friendship Publishing Co. ISBN: 7505721607. 2006-4-1

Brief Biography of Lu: Liu Shun born in Hubei Province (1363–1489), died at the age of 126 years old. He was given a royal mandate to setup clinical experimentation for cancer on death-row inmates. After 66 years of cancer research, he summarized a set of cancer prevention guidelines: 30% Medication and 70% Nourishment Which became the standard TCM treatment protocol. His motto: "When a person lacks the stomach Qi, the digestive capability, then medicine is useless. Rather starve to death than be poisoned to death (the side-effect of toxic herbs). Rather die like a fool, than die from irritation; Rather die of exhaustion, than to die from idleness." 刘家高祖刘纯，字景厚，号养正老人；湖北省咸宁人。生于公元1363 年，卒于公1489 年，享年126 岁。他是刘完素的九世孙，被明清两朝太医院尊为太医保护神。他奉旨以囚试医，带领

医 官经过66 年的努力，总结出一套预防疾病的养生十条，和治疗疾病的生饥、食疗、慎用药的三分治 七分养方法，使得后世受益无穷。他的遗训： "人无胃气不治,药不亲尝不发" ，以及 "宁可饿死,切勿毒死;宁可傻死,切勿气死;宁可累死,切勿闲死。" 也是刘家的座右铭。

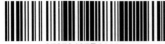

Made in the USA
Columbia, SC
23 September 2018